LASER VISION CORRECTION

D.

Copyright © 2009 E.E. Anderson Penno, M.D.
All rights reserved.

Some images reprinted with permission from
Abbott Medical Optics, Santa Ana, CA.

ISBN: 1-4392-6497-X
EAN13: 9781439264973

To my family for their love and support.

INTRODUCTION

Recently a patient inquired about laser eye surgery saying, "I've been to three different laser centers and was told something different at each one. How do I know which surgery is the best?" I realized that the answer is more complicated than can be covered completely during a short clinic visit. It is also challenging to find a single up to date source for concise, accurate information intended for the consumer. This book was created for consumers that may not have a medical or scientific background who are trying to decide if they should undergo laser vision correction.

The information in this book is not a substitute for a surgeon's opinion, but will help provide basic information about the options available for laser vision correction surgery. Be sure to talk to your eye care provider about any questions you have, and ask if there are new technologic developments. The more knowledge you have, the more confident you will be in your choices about laser vision correction.

TABLE OF CONTENTS

PART I: BASIC FACTS 3

Chapter 1: Laser Vision Correction Essentials 5
Chapter 2: What is far-sighted, near-sighted,
            and astigmatism? 23
Chapter 3: Who is a Candidate for Laser Vision
            Correction? 35
Chapter 4: How to Choose a Surgeon 53
Chapter 5: How to Choose Between PRK, LASIK, Epi-LASIK &
            Intra-LASIK 69
Chapter 6: What to Expect from Laser
            Vision Correction 83

PART II: LASER VISION CORRECTION IN DETAIL 97

Chapter 7:   Eye Anatomy 99
Chapter 8:   PRK: Photorefractive Keratectomy 121
Chapter 9:   Epi-LASIK 133
Chapter 10: LASIK: Laser in situ Keratomeleusis 145
Chapter 11: Intra-LASIK 157
Chapter 12: Laser Types: Wavefront/Custom/
             Aspheric Ablation 167
Chapter 13: Alternate (non-laser) Vision
             Correction Options 173

Resources 179
Glossary 181

PART I: **BASIC FACTS**

CHAPTER 1: LASER VISION CORRECTION ESSENTIALS

This chapter is designed to cover basic facts that anyone considering laser vision correction should know. It is important to make sure these facts are well understood prior to undergoing laser vision correction. Once a decision is made as to which type of surgery will be performed, the details of that specific procedure should also be well understood in order for you to make a good decision regarding risks and benefits. Having the right expectations will make it more likely that you will be happy with the results of laser vision correction.

Although the success rate of currently available vision correction surgeries is quite good, the risk is very real. If you were among the less than one percent of people who have serious complications following laser vision correction, would you be able to cope with a permanent reduction of acuity in one or both eyes? Consider your options carefully to determine what level of risk you may be willing to take in order to have benefits such as more rapid recovery of vision and less discomfort.

The details can be overwhelming, but it is well worth the time spent to fully understand the choices you are making when selecting a surgeon and type of vision correction surgery. It is important to read all materials including surgical consent forms that may be given to you by your surgeon. Be sure to have all your questions answered before undergoing any type of laser vision correction surgery.

What is laser vision correction?

Laser vision correction refers to any surgical procedure that uses an excimer laser to reshape the cornea (please refer to Chapter 7 for basic anatomy of the eye). The cornea is the clear surface on the front of the eye through which you can see the iris (colored part of the eye) and the pupil.

The laser is used to vaporize the tissue in a precise pattern which reshapes the corneal surface such that dependence on glasses or contact lenses is reduced or eliminated. This process of vaporizing corneal tissue by the excimer laser is called ablation.

The surgeon who performs the procedure is an ophthalmologist who is a medical doctor (MD) with a specialty in the diagnosis of eye disease, treatment of eye disease, and eye surgery. The surgeon should be board certified. A surgeon who is board certified in the United States is designated as a Diplomate American Board of Ophthalmology (Dipl. ABO) and in Canada as a Fellow of the Royal College of Surgeons of Canada (FRCSC). There are often optometrists who work in association with an ophthalmologist who may do the initial assessment at some centers. Other staff such as technicians will also participate in your care.

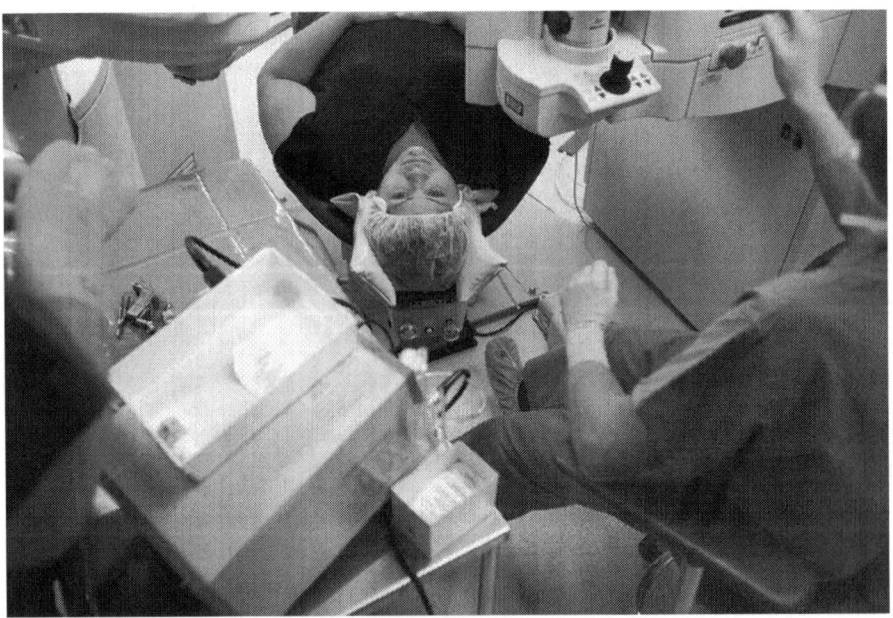

Chapter 1: Laser Vision Correction Essentials

The types of staff involved in your care may include:

Ophthalmologist (MD):	medical doctor specialized in eye care and eye surgery
Optometrist (OD):	doctor of optometry trained in medical eye care
Certified Ophthalmic Medical Technologist (COMT):	the highest technician designation that assistants in eye care can achieve through the Joint Commission on Allied Health Personnel in Ophthalmology (JCAHPO)
Certified Ophthalmic Technician (COT):	second highest level of JCAHPO certification held by assisting staff
Certified Ophthalmic Assistant (COA):	first level of certification available to eye care assistants through JCAHPO
Counselors:	staff specializing in giving detailed information to patients.
Receptionist:	staff who will be involved in scheduling appointments.

Pay attention to the quality of the front office staff including reception and secretaries. A well run center should have prompt and courteous care starting from your initial telephone inquiry and throughout your visits. If you choose to undergo surgery you will be spending time with a variety of staff members during your testing, counseling, surgery, and post-operative care.

Laser vision correction is also called refractive surgery or laser eye surgery. The procedures can be divided into two groups: those with flaps and those without flaps.

The most commonly available specific types of surgeries are:

Photorefractive keratectomy (PRK):	the original no-flap surgery introduced in the US in 1988 by Margueritte MacDonald.
Epi-LASIK:	the latest no-flap procedure in which an epikeratome is used to remove the outer epithelial layer to prepare for laser application.
Laser in situ Keratomeleusis (LASIK):	the first flap procedure introduced in the 1990s in which uses a mechanical microkeratome to create a flap.
Intra-LASIK:	a newer flap procedure which uses a femtosecond laser to create a flap.

The details of these procedures are covered in depth in Part II of this book.

For PRK and Epi-LASIK the surface corneal epithelial cells are removed and the laser is applied directly to the corneal surface. For PRK the surface cells can be removed using dilute alcohol or with a brush. For Epi-LASIK an automated device called an epikeratome is used to remove the surface cells to prepare the corneal surface for the laser reshaping.

PRK has been around for over two decades and has an excellent long term safety record. Epi-LASIK is a newer technique that creates a precise epithelial removal that will help speed recovery. Because there is no flap to protect the surface while healing, PRK and Epi-LASIK result in more discomfort for the first few days after surgery and take four to ten days before the vision is recovered enough to resume driving and/or work. Medicated drops may be recommended a few times per day for a number of weeks or months after surgery. The long term vision results are excellent. The simplicity of the surgical technique means there is a lower chance of complications during surgery and no flap that could become damaged or dislodged due to injury in the future. Recently many surgeons have returned to PRK and Epi-LASIK as their recommended vision correction surgery due to the low rate of complications.

With LASIK and Intra-LASIK a corneal flap is created and the laser treatment is applied to the bed of tissue under the flap. LASIK was developed in the 1990s. LASIK is a combination of an older technique called lamellar keratoplasty in which a corneal flap was created and PRK. It has been called "flap and zap" in the past. For LASIK a mechanical device called a microkeratome is used to create a corneal flap. Flaps can range in thickness from 90 microns to 180 microns depending on the device used. For Intra-LASIK an ultrafast femtosecond laser is used to create the flaps.

Vision recovery following a flap procedure is quicker than with a surface treatment. In an uncomplicated case the patient may expect some discomfort and blurred vision for the first twenty-four hours. By the following day in most cases patients will be legal to drive, although there is long term healing that will be occurring so some patients may find the vision continues to sharpen for a number of days to weeks. There is a higher risk with flap procedures due to the complexity of creating the flap and the possibility that the flap could become damaged or shifted if a future eye injury occurs. In rare cases flaps may be shifted even months or years later. In most cases common sense eye safety should protect you from this type of injury. However, if you are in a high risk occupation or have high risk hobbies PRK or Epi-LASIK may be a better choice. Although higher risk, some consumers will opt for LASIK or Intra-LASIK due to the shorter recovery.

There may be reasons why a specific type of vision correction surgery may be recommended as safest for your individual case. Alternatively you may be given a choice of procedures, in which case you will need to weigh the risks and benefits of each procedure to make the choice that is right for you.

What is an excimer laser?

The excimer laser uses argon and fluorine gases to create laser energy with a wavelength of 193 nm. This wavelength is very specific to corneal tissue and allows for the precise ablation (evaporation) of corneal tissue. Avco Everett Research Laboratories and the United States Government Laboratories played an important role in developing the excimer technology in the 1970s. Excimer technology was invented by a number of scientists including Trokel and Srinavasin who introduced the excimer laser for corneal refractive surgery in 1983. The US FDA approved PRK in 1995.

Many people give Dr. Pallikaris credit for creating LASIK in the 1990s. LASIK was a combination of prior corneal flap making techniques with PRK. Called "flap and zap" by some providers LASIK quickly became popular in the 1990s. A renewed interest in surface no flap techniques has occurred recently with Epi-LASIK developing over the past few years. The femtosecond laser has recently been introduced as a safer flap making technique.

In spite of these advances, PRK still remains a good choice for a simple and reliable technique for laser vision correction. The differences include different risks of each type of surgery, differences in the first few days in terms of vision and comfort, and differences in the first weeks in terms of vision recovery. The long term results of all of the laser vision correction techniques are similar.

Who is eligible for laser vision correction?

During the assessment there are a number of things the surgeon will be looking at to determine whether or not you qualify for laser vision correction. There are corneal con-

Chapter 1: Laser Vision Correction Essentials

ditions such as irregularity of the corneal surface or thin corneas that you may not be aware of prior to your preoperative assessment that may disqualify you from laser vision correction. There are also some medical conditions that may increase your risks or affect your outcomes. Finally, very high corrections may not be suitable for laser vision correction. There are also a variety of conditions that may make you more susceptible to long term post-operative side effects.

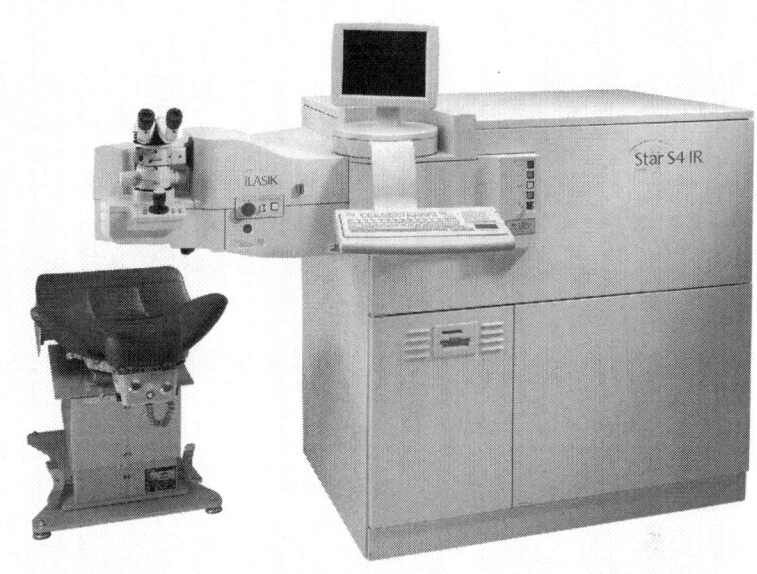

The excimer laser is used to precisely reshape the cornea during laser vision correction surgery.

The basic requirements are:

Age:	you must be over the age of eighteen.
Stability:	you must have a stable vision correction for one to two years.
Eye health:	you must be free from serious eye disease.
Corneal thickness:	the corneas must be thick enough to support the treatment.
Prescription:	extremely high or very low corrections may not qualify.

More information on what factors are considered to determine if you qualify for laser vision correction can be found in Chapter 3.

Why do I have to leave my contact lenses out before assessment and surgery?

Most people who wear contact lenses full time do not like to wear their glasses. It may be less frustrating to wear your glasses for a period of time if you understand why you are instructed to leave your contacts out.

Contact lens wear can warp the corneal surface and in some people will lead to chronic dry eye. These surface changes can affect the testing, including the corneal mapping results. In some cases, if the mapping is abnormal, your eye care provider may ask you to leave contacts out for a longer period of time and suggest dry eye treatments to optimize mapping results. Corneal mapping is done to identify people who may have a high risk for corneal instability, also called ectasia, following laser vision correction.

For true wavefront treatments soft lenses may need to be left out for one to two weeks. This is especially important for wavefront treatments since the measurements of higher levels of irregularity (higher order aberrations) will be used to create the individualized laser treatment plan. Rigid gas permeable lenses may need to be left out for a longer period of time for the cornea the return to its natural state.

Even if you choose not to have laser vision correction it is wise to have a current pair of glasses for back up. There may be reasons such as infection or injury that may require you to be out of your contacts, in some cases for several weeks or months. In these situations it can be challenging to get an accurate new prescription, and having a current pair of eye glasses will help you remain functional until contacts can be safely worn again.

What should I expect from laser vision correction?

The goal of laser vision correction should be for you to function as well without glasses for distance as you do now with your corrective lenses. The laser treatment is intended to bring your prescription to zero for distance. This means that if you are able to see 20/20 with your corrective lenses, you will be likely to achieve 20/20 for distance after laser vision correction. A measurement of 20/20 is considered normal vision and means that you can see at 20 feet a specific line on a standard Snellen eye chart. Some people can see a little better than 20/20, such as 20/15 or rarely 20/10. The metric equivalent of 20/20 is 6/6 which refers to vision measured at 6 meters. If you are unable to see 20/20 with corrective lenses in one or both eyes you are likely to have the same vision after laser vision correction that you do with your most up to date eyewear. There is a more in depth discussion of visual acuity in Chapter 7.

If you are over the age of forty or are already wearing progressive or bifocal lenses, you can expect to need reading glasses either immediately after surgery or within a few years. Even people who do not wear glasses for distance (either because they never needed them or because they had laser vision correction) will need reading glasses by about age 45. The only way to reduce dependence on reading glasses is to leave one eye undercorrected or nearsighted for reading. This is called mono-vision and will be discussed in more detail in Chapters 2 and 3. For those considering laser vision correction at a younger age, you also will need readers once you reach your fourth decade. At this time there is no way to correct the loss of focus that occurs as a natural consequence of aging.

It may not be possible for you to see exactly as sharply as you do with your current lenses. If you wear gas permeable lenses you may find that the vision may not be quite as crisp after surgery. There is some evidence that a true customized laser pattern, also called wavefront, may improve visual outcomes. This will be discussed in more detail in Chapter 12.

Most surgeons will tell you that the expectation should be to see as well as you do at the distance now with your corrective lenses, not better. The same is true for night vision. For the first few weeks or months after surgery you may experience glare or halo at night. Most people will find that after several weeks or months their night vision is similar to what they had prior to surgery. This means if you don't like to drive at night before vision correction surgery you probably still won't like driving at night. If you are very particular about your vision you should carefully consider the risk that your quality of vision may be reduced as a result of surgery.

Those who have dry eyes before surgery with contact lenses may find their eyes temporarily even more dry after surgery and will likely always have a dry eye after surgery. Those who do not wear contacts due to dry eye may find a permanent worsening of dry eye after surgery due to the fact that glasses provide a good vapor barrier to prevent evaporation and protect the eyes from wind or dust. After surgery the eyes will no longer have the protection of glasses unless you choose to wear sunglasses or clear lenses. Many people find their eyes are permanently a little more sensitive to irritants like smoke once they do not have glasses or contacts to provide a barrier to these irritants.

Chapter 1: Laser Vision Correction Essentials

A certain percentage of people will need a second laser treatment for their best vision. This is called an enhancement, retreatment, or a touch-up. This is not considered a complication but rather a consequence of the fact that each cornea has individual biologic factors that will cause the tissue to respond or heal slightly differently from person to person. The higher the correction, the more likely that a second treatment may be needed.

Farsighted corrections may also have a higher likelihood of needing an enhancement. The surgeon may choose to wait up to six months or longer before recommending a touch-up as the correction in some people may take longer to stabilize. A few patients may need interim glasses while they are waiting for stabilization. If an enhancement is necessary it will usually be needed within the first year. In general the distance correction should be stable for a number of years following laser vision correction surgery unless other conditions develop such as cataract which can cause a shift in the correction.

For uncomplicated laser vision correction surgery there are some conditions that you may experience after surgery:

The most common permanent side effects are:

Dry eye:	most common if your eyes are dry before surgery. Many people are more sensitive the airborne irritants like smoke.
Glare and halo:	this can affect night vision especially in very high corrections.
Reading glasses:	will be needed for those near or in their forties or older.

These side effects do not affect everyone. Your surgeon should discuss with you any factors that put you at a high risk for these or other complications. If there is a complication of surgery there may be a loss of vision that may or may not be correctable with glasses or contact lenses or that may require additional surgery.

Why is the pricing so different between centers?

Laser vision correction centers are businesses. Just as different retail chains offer different levels of service and products, laser vision correction centers vary in their business models. Some do higher volumes and have many centers so can benefit from volume pricing on surgical supplies, and they pass that savings to their clients. Some centers offer more individualized care with the surgeon before and after surgery such that lower volumes of patients are being treated but at a higher price.

Pricing can also be difficult to judge at first glance. Sometimes the advertised low price may only apply to very simple corrections and may not include enhancements. When searching for the right center to have vision correction surgery, it is wise to shop around to find the combination of price and service that fits you best. Be sure to find out what is included in the base price and who will be providing your pre- and post-procedure care.

Pricing not only will vary between centers, and it will also likely vary between procedures. For example, a standard laser treatment may be less expensive than a custom wavefront treatment due to the costs of providing the custom treatment. Some centers may have different prices for PRK, Epi-LASIK, LASIK, and Intra-LASIK due to the costs associated with providing each of the different procedures. Some centers have different pricing for different levels of correction such that higher corrections may pay more than lower corrections.

Price is an important factor but should not overshadow safety, effectiveness, and the level of service that you may need as an individual. As in all other consumer services you can not judge on price alone. Each individual needs to weigh the price and levels of service offered by the various centers and decide which one is right for them.

Questions you may wish to ask about pricing include:

1. What are the prices for the surgeries you are considering for your individual case? Some centers use a price scale based on your level of correction.
2. Does the price include enhancements (touch up surgery) and for how long?
3. Are all the pre-operative and post-operative visits included in the price?
4. Are there payment plans available?
5. Can the center provide documentation for spending accounts or insurance if needed?

What to consider when choosing a laser vision correction center & surgeon

Many centers will offer a free assessment. Although time consuming, it may be helpful to go through assessments at different centers in order to learn about the services they offer and get an individualized quote for your case. Once you have been identified as a suitable candidate you should educate yourself by asking a lot of questions.

Questions to ask once you are told you are a candidate for surgery:

1. If a specific procedure is recommended, why was that recommendation made?
2. Do you have a choice of procedures and what are pros/cons of each?
3. How many of that procedure has the surgeon done?
4. What are the surgeon's credentials?
5. How long has the surgeon been at the center?
6. If you didn't meet the surgeon at the assessment, when will you meet?
7. What is the complication rate of that procedure with that particular surgeon?

8. What should I expect during and after surgery?
9. Who will be providing my post-operative care?
10. What is the chance that an enhancement will be needed?
11. Is there anything unique about my case?
12. Is the surgeon local? Some surgeons travel from elsewhere to do surgery.
13. If my surgeon doesn't reside locally, is there a covering surgeon on location?

Be sure to add questions as you learn more about laser vision correction and read all informational materials supplied to you including surgical consent.

It is helpful to talk to friends and family about their experiences, although keep in mind that each individual case is different so their experiences may not always apply to you. If you have an eye care provider such as an optometrist or ophthalmologist it can be very helpful to discuss with that provider your particular suitability for vision correction, who they may recommend, and why they would recommend a particular surgeon. In some cases your regular eye care provider may be able to co-manage your care prior to and after surgery.

It is important to understand that although the risk is low, if you have a complication from surgery you may need to work closely with the surgeon and laser center staff over a number of weeks or months to correct a problem. The vast majority of patients do very well and need only a few visits before and after surgery. However, if you are a higher risk candidate or do suffer a complication you will want to be in good hands.

What if there is a complication?

The complication rates for vision correction surgery are very low. Requiring a second treatment or enhancement is not considered to be a complication as a certain percentage of patients will be expected to return for touch-up due to biologic differences in healing and response to the laser.

Complications are generally divided into the following categories:

Intra-operative Complications: problems that happen during the surgery.

Early Post-operative Complications: problems within a few days after surgery.

Late Post-operative Complications: problems occurring after months or years.

The main goal of the assessment before surgery is to identify things that might put you at a higher risk for any complications during or after laser vision correction. It is not possible for any surgeon to predict all complications, but the goal is to minimize the risks of laser vision correction by doing a thorough assessment before deciding if it is safe to proceed.

The most common type of complication would be something that may delay healing or require additional medications to correct. In more rare cases a serious complication may occur which could require additional surgeries to correct. In very rare cases there could be a complication that may not be correctable and that may lead to a permanent loss of sight. This risk is low but it is not zero.

In order to insure that you understand the risks and benefits of a laser vision correction procedure you will be asked to read and sign a consent for that procedure. The surgeon will also sign to indicate that you have had a chance to discuss the risks and benefits of the procedure. By signing the consent you are confirming that you have read and understood the document, and that you have asked any questions you may have about the risks and benefits. By educating yourself prior to and throughout the assessment process you will feel more confident in your choices for laser vision correction.

Where to find additional information

There are several sources of information available to learn about laser vision correction surgeries. A good place to start is with your current eye care provider. Your optometrist or ophthalmologist will very likely be familiar with what is available in your area even if they aren't affiliated with a laser vision correction center. In addition, if you have been with that provider for a number of visits they may be able to tell you if you may be a good basic candidate for surgery. Of course additional tests will need to be performed during a laser vision assessment to confirm that you qualify for surgery.

Friends and family that have undergone surgery can give you information about a particular center in terms of how their individual case was handled. Keep in mind that a single poor outcome does not necessarily mean the center or the surgeon was at fault. However, complaints about service from multiple people may be a red flag.

There are a few books and articles available ranging from general information to more specific topics. When reading material be aware that there may be changes in technology over time. General surgical principles may remain constant, but if a book or article is more than about three years old there may be new technologies available. On the other hand there are techniques such as PRK which have withstood the test of time. The basic techniques of PRK have undergone some changes over the years, but the major change to PRK is in the laser application with the introduction of sophisticated techniques such as wavefront treatments. In order to understand both the old and the new it is helpful to read current material.

The internet is the venue of choice for most people when they are first researching a topic. It is especially important on the web to consider the source of information as far as accuracy of information.

Reliable Internet Information on Laser Vision Correction

Mayoclinic.com:	website for the Mayo Clinic
AAO.org:	American Academy of Ophthalmology
ASCRS.org:	American Society of Cataract and Refractive Surgery
Ncbi.nlm.nih.gov/pubmed:	US National Library of Medicine and the National Institute of Health peer reviewed articles

It may also be helpful to look on the website of the center where you are considering laser vision correction surgery.

Summary

To navigate the complexities of laser vision correction surgery you will need to take advantage off all resources available including your current eye care provider, trusted internet sites, books, and staff and surgeons at laser vision correction centers. Details of specific laser vision correction surgeries can be found in Part II of this book. If you are not a candidate for laser vision correction or are interested in alternatives the non-laser options are discussed in Chapter 13.

CHAPTER 2: WHAT IS FARSIGHTED, NEARSIGHTED, AND ASTIGMATISM?

The need for corrective lenses is called "refractive error". For this reason laser vision correction is also known as "refractive surgery". The refraction describes the optical state of the eye without any lenses.

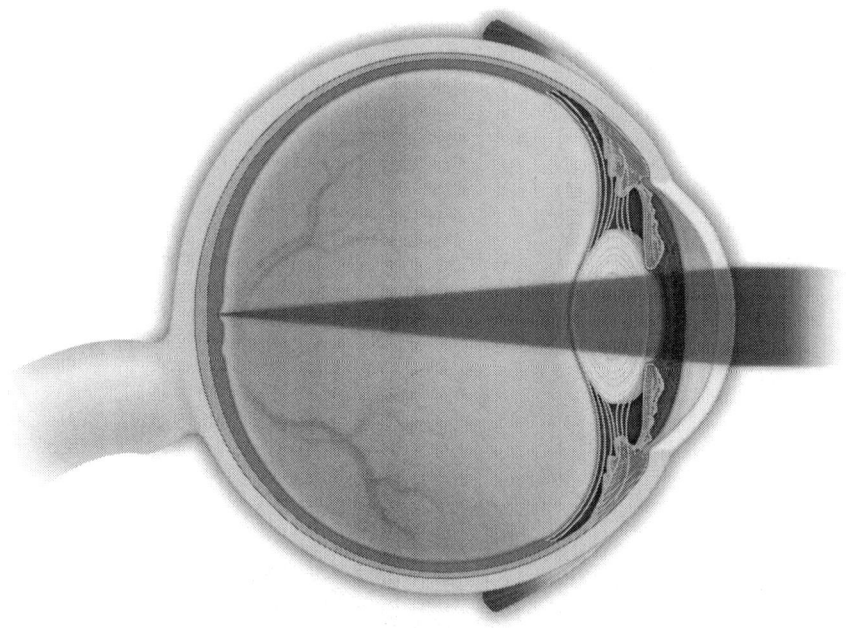

Light entering an eye that does not require corrective lenses comes to a focal point on the retina.

Types of Refractive Errors

Nearsighted (myopia): a nearsighted or myopic eye has a focal point closer than infinity. The higher the myopia the closer the focal point.

Farsighted (hyperopia): the farsighted or hyperopic eye has a focal point beyond infinity such that the eye must exert focal power to see clearly even at distance.

Astigmatism: in most cases astigmatism results from a cornea that is shaped more like a football than a basketball. Corrective lenses with astigmatism correction compensate for this non-spherical shape.

Presbyopia: presbyopia is the loss of focus power which is a natural part of the aging process. Presbyopia happens to everyone and results in the need for reading glasses, bifocal or progressive lenses, or taking your glasses off to read by the time you are in your mid to late forties.

The measurement of your prescription is called a refraction. During the refraction you will be shown a series of lenses and asked to choose between various lenses. People who wear glasses are very familiar with the question the examiner will ask when showing lenses, "Which is better one or two?" Since this choice is subjective, there may be minor variations in the prescriptions between tests. There are different ways to measure the refractive error.

Chapter 2: What is Farsighted, Nearsighted, and Astigmatism?

Measurements of Refractive Error

Manifest refraction: also known as a "dry refraction", the manifest refraction is done without the use of eye drops. This is the most common method.

Cycloplegic refraction: also known as a "wet refraction", the cycloplegic refraction is done after dilation drops are used to relax the focus power of the eye.

Auto-refraction: this method uses an automated device to estimate the refraction.

Wavefront refraction: this method uses an infrared technique combined with an aberrometer (sophisticated device that measures individual variations of the eye).

During the pre-operative assessment you will most likely have the manifest, cycloplegic, and auto-refraction measured. If your surgeon uses wavefront technology then you will also have the wavefront refraction measured. The surgeon will consider all of the measurements along with the measurements of your current lenses and any past information available to determine if your correction is stable. All of this information is taken into consideration when determining what data is entered into the laser for treatment.

Nearsighted (Myopia)

Myopia is the technical term for nearsightedness. Myopia can run in families. People who are myopic (nearsighted) can not see far distance without corrective lenses. The higher the correction, the closer the focal point. This relationship is known as Snell's law.

The nearsighted eye is either too long or has a cornea that is too steep. This results in light coming to a focal point inside the eye in front of the retina. To focus the light onto the retina an object has to be brought closer to the eye or the nearsightedness needs to be corrected with glasses or contact lenses.

The earlier the age that a person needs a nearsighted correction, the higher the eventual correction. There have been many studies over the years that suggest that excessive near work may lead to increasing nearsightedness, although the link between near work myopia has not been proven. Recently researchers have studied time spent

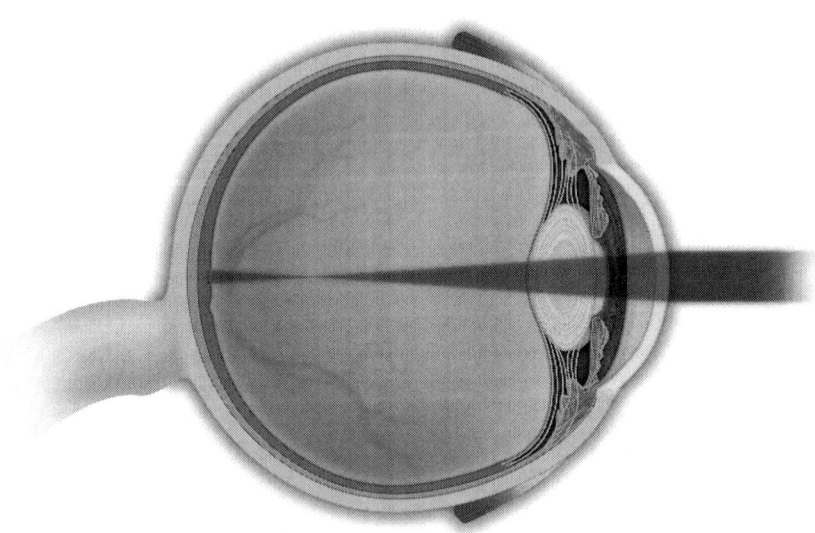

Light entering a nearsighted eye comes to a focal before it reaches the retina.

Chapter 2: What is Farsighted, Nearsighted, and Astigmatism?

outdoors and suggest that children who spend more time outdoors may be less likely to become nearsighted.

In general nearsightedness will continue to progress through the teen years and stabilize around age eighteen to twenty in a low correction. For high corrections the prescription may not stabilize until the mid-twenties to thirties. In pathologic myopia or extreme nearsightedness the eye will continue to progress to a higher correction through-out life. Pathologic myopia will often have corrections of fifteen to twenty diopters or higher.

It is important to have a stable prescription for at least one year and preferably two or three years before having laser vision correction. When the eye is naturally becoming more nearsighted with age it is called progression. Laser vision correction will not stop progression so if a treatment is done before the eye is stable then the nearsightedness will return over months to years.

When the glasses check or refraction is done it is possible for the examiner to give more correction than is really needed due to the focusing ability of the eye. This is called over-minusing. If your correction has crept up a quarter or half of a diopter over a few years it is possible that your prescription may be stronger than you need. For this reason a cycloplegic refraction or a glasses check after dilation drops is done before laser vision correction surgery. The cycloplegic refraction will relax the focus ability of the eye and can identify when a person has been over-minused.

The excimer laser is used to flatten the cornea for a nearsighted correction. The resulting flatter cornea is able to push the focal point of light further back onto the retina and in that way provides better uncorrected vision. The higher the correction the more corneal tissue has to be removed. For this reason very high corrections may result in over thinning of the cornea which leads to corneal instability or ectasia. Part of the pre-operative assessment is to determine if the cornea is thick enough to support treatment of the specific amount of nearsightedness.

Farsighted (Hyperopia)

The farsighted eye is also known as hyperopic. In the fully relaxed farsighted eye, light from a distance comes to a focal point behind the eye. In order for an object to be brought into focus in the fully relaxed farsighted eye the object would have to be moved beyond infinity. A farsighted or hyperopic eye is too short or the cornea is too flat.

For younger patients with lower amounts of farsightedness the ability to focus or accommodate will bring an object at both near and distance into focus until they are in their twenties or thirties. In these cases reading glasses may be needed at a younger age, sometimes in the twenties or thirties. For lower amounts of farsightedness a distance correction will also become necessary in the thirties, forties, or fifties. This is known as "latent hyperopia".

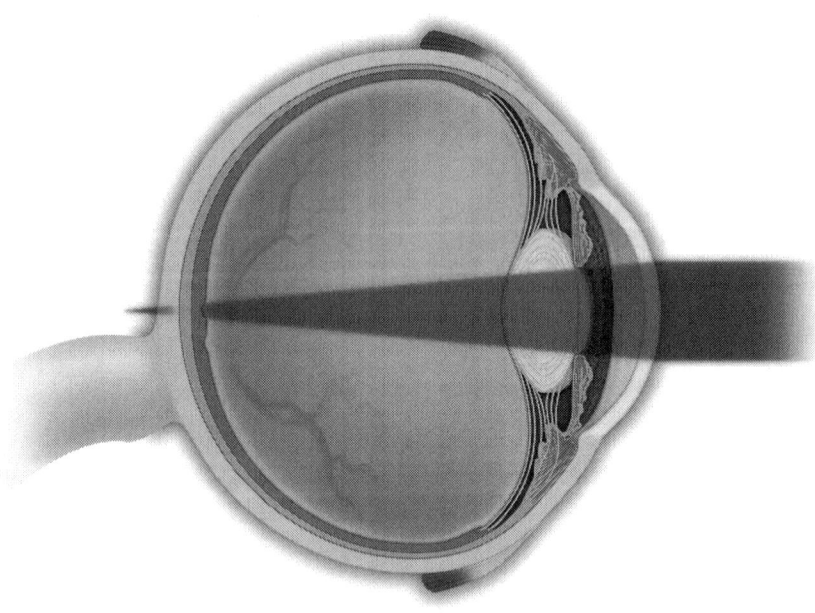

Light entering a farsighted eye will come to a focal point beyond the retina.

Chapter 2: What is Farsighted, Nearsighted, and Astigmatism?

For higher amounts of farsightedness corrective lenses for both distance and close may be needed at a younger age. Eventually for both high and low hyperopia, a bifocal or progressive lens will be needed to correct for reading vision sometime after age forty. The cycloplegic refraction can determine the true amount of farsightedness at any age because it will temporarily relax the focusing ability of the eye.

To correct farsightedness the cornea is made steeper by removing more tissue from the peripheral (outer edges) cornea than the center. Due to the shape that results from farsighted laser vision correction, there is more likelihood of regression. Regression is a healing response that shifts the eye back towards the original correction. The resulting shape also means that higher farsighted corrections may have poorer optical quality.

During the pre-operative testing a cycloplegic refraction must be done to determine the true amount of farsightedness, otherwise it is likely there will be an under-correction with a need for distance glasses in the future as the age related loss of focus ability occurs. If you are farsighted you should be sure to understand this relationship between your prescription, your age, and your focusing ability in order to make a good choice as to whether laser vision correction is right for you.

Astigmatism

Regular astigmatism occurs most often when the cornea is shaped more like a football than a basketball. In other words, when the cornea is not a perfect sphere there is a refractive error present which is called astigmatism. Astigmatism can also result from an optical variation in the lens of the eye. The measurement of astigmatism will consist of an amount and an axis. A good analogy is how steep the football is and how it is rotated. The football will be lying flat or standing vertical or tilted somewhere in between.

Regular astigmatism can be corrected with glasses or contact lenses. A lens that contains an astigmatism correction is called a toric lens.

Irregular astigmatism can result from corneal scars or other corneal injury. Using the analogy of the football, in irregular astigmatism the football may be partly deflated with folds in it or may have extra lumps or bumps on the surface such that there are not smooth regular curves. Irregular astigmatism can not be corrected with glasses. In some cases irregular astigmatism can be corrected by contact lenses. In some cases specialized contact lenses are needed to correct irregular astigmatism. In severe cases of irregular astigmatism due to corneal disease a corneal transplant may be necessary.

Regular astigmatism can be present in combination with nearsightedness or farsightedness. If the prescription is stable, regular astigmatism can be treated with laser vision correction. Extremely high amounts of astigmatism may not respond well to laser vision correction. In some cases high astigmatism might be present in cases of corneal dystrophy such as keratoconus. As part of the assessment a corneal map will be done which can show if the astigmatism is regular and if there are signs of keratoconus or other corneal dystrophy.

If you have astigmatism you should talk to your surgeon about your chances of needing an enhancement. Higher astigmatism can be associated with a higher need for retreatment or enhancement. In cases of high astigmatism the surgeon may choose to mark the cornea at the slit lamp prior to treatment to make sure the eye is aligned properly with respect to rotation. There are some lasers with the ability to recognize the iris and make a cyclotorsion (rotational) adjustment for better accuracy in treatment of astigmatism. As with any refractive error your prescription should be stable before considering laser vision correction.

Chapter 2: What is Farsighted, Nearsighted, and Astigmatism?

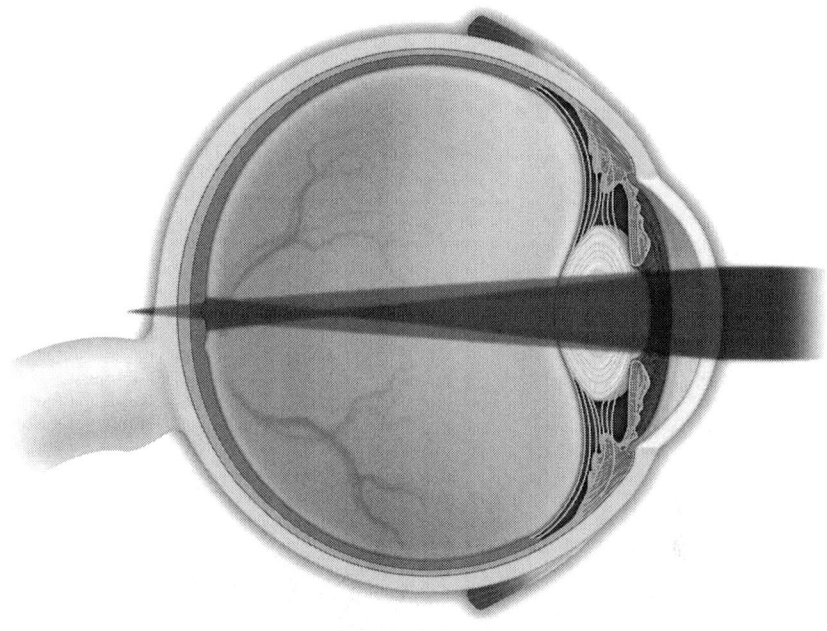

Light entering an eye with astigmatism has two different focal points.

Laser Vision Correction

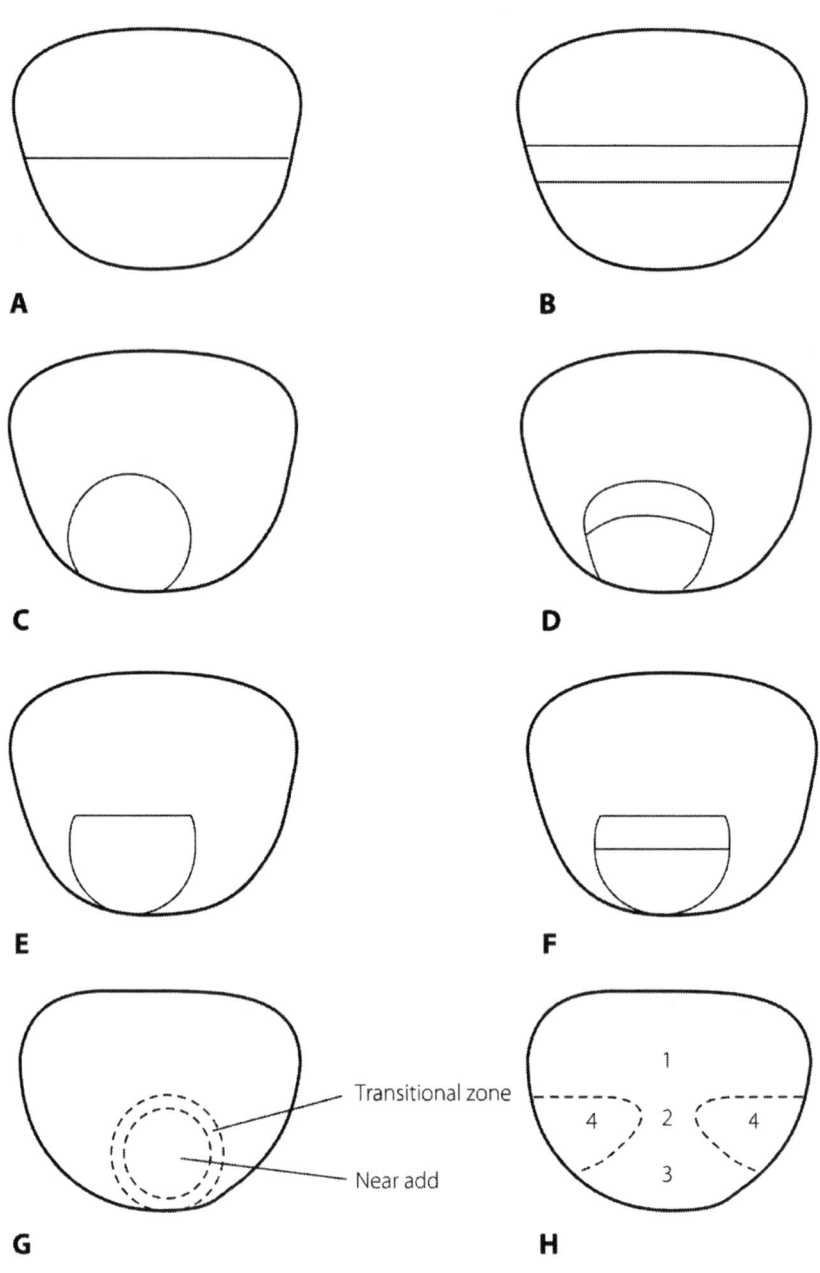

After the age of 40 a bifocal, trifocal, or other type of multifocal correction will be needed to maintain the ability to read with distance glasses on. © 2009 American Academy of Ophthalmology

Chapter 2: What is Farsighted, Nearsighted, and Astigmatism?

Presbyopia

As a natural part of the aging process the focusing ability of the eye will weaken. For most people this will result in the need for reading glasses or a bifocal between the ages of forty and forty-five.

Presbyopia Correction

Reading glasses: those who don't need glasses for distance or for people who wear contact lenses for distance, reading glasses will be needed after age forty.

Bifocal glasses: for those who need glasses for distance, a bifocal lens will be needed; a bifocal has a visible reading segment in the eyeglass.

Progressive glasses: progressive lenses have a reading segment in the lower part of the glass; progressive lenses are also known as "lineless bifocals".

Monovision: some mildly nearsighted people will wear a contact lens in one eye only; or for higher corrections one eye will be corrected for near vision.

Bifocal contacts: bifocal and multifocal contact lenses are also available.

Taking glasses off: mildly nearsighted people sometimes simply take their glasses off to read.

Multifocal lens implants: if you are over the age of 55 and/or have cataracts, a multifocal lens implant may restore some of your close vision.

If you are approaching or over the age of forty you should be sure to speak to your surgeon about the need for reading glasses or bifocals. For farsighted people, reading glasses may be needed at a younger age. Underestimating the need for reading glasses is one of the most common reasons that people in this age range are unhappy with laser vision correction. If you are mildly nearsighted and take your glasses off to read, you will be trading reading glasses for your current distance correction.

Summary

Farsightedness, astigmatism, and nearsightedness can all be corrected by laser vision correction. It is important to understand your individual prescription and the effect of age on your focusing ability, and to discuss how it may affect your suitability for laser vision correction.

CHAPTER 3: WHO IS A CANDIDATE FOR LASER VISION CORRECTION?

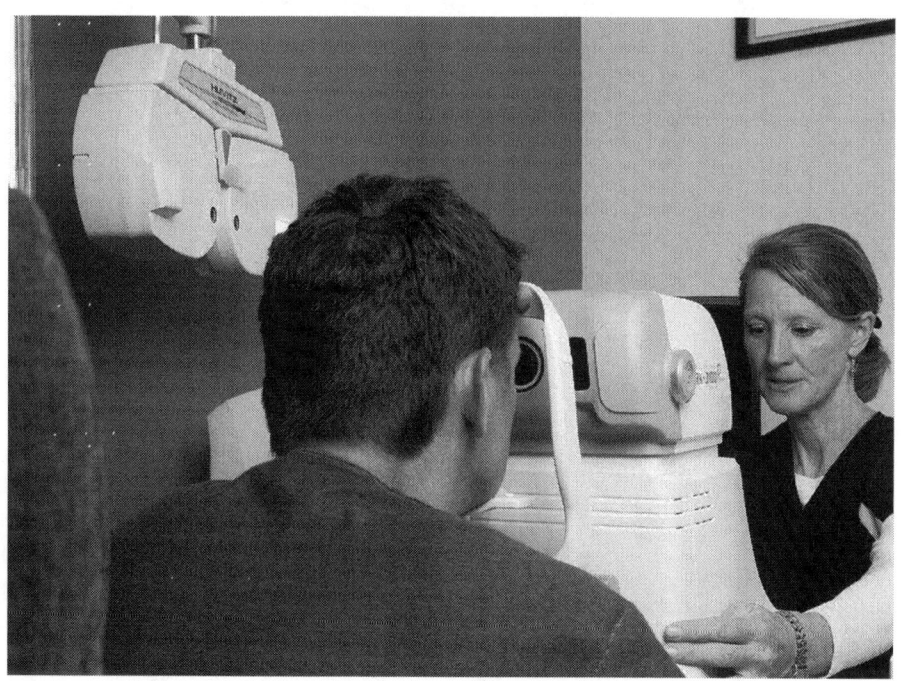

Photo by Dave Best.

About twenty-five percent of people who undergo a laser vision correction assessment will not be candidates for surgery. There are a number of things that may disqualify you from laser vision correction. There are some factors such as thin corneas which may disqualify you for deeper treatments like LASIK or Intra-LASIK but may not disqualify you for surface treatments like PRK and Epi-LASIK.

Your assessment should include a complete history including eye history, medical history, family history of eye disease, eye medications, general medications, and allergies. The assessment will also include a complete dilated eye examination with refraction (checking the eyeglass correction), corneal thickness measurements, and corneal mapping. There may be additional tests performed such as measurements of tear production or field of vision if the examining doctor feels these tests are needed.

This chapter will include the most common factors to be considered when determining candidacy for laser vision correction.

Factors for determining candidacy include:

Age:	at least eighteen years old and usually younger than fifty-five.
Occupation:	factors such as risk of trauma and vision requirements.
Hobbies:	requirements for distance or close vision will be considered.
Refraction (nearsighted, farsighted, astigmatism):	too high or too low.
Refraction stability:	stability for at least one to two years is required.
Corneal thickness:	must be thick enough to undergo surgery.
Corneal maps:	pattern must not show signs of corneal disorder.
Eye health:	you must be free from serious eye disease.
Family history:	family history of corneal disease may disqualify you.
Medical history:	some conditions will rule out laser vision correction.
Expectations:	realistic expectations are critical for laser vision correction.

Chapter 3: Who is a Candidate for Laser Vision Correction?

There may be reasons that are not discussed in this chapter why you may not qualify for laser vision correction. Your surgeon should discuss with you what factors may disqualify you or may put you at higher risk for complication from laser vision correction.

Age

The minimum age for laser vision correction is usually considered to be eighteen years. While there is no absolute maximum, most surgeons will hesitate to perform laser vision correction over the age of fifty-five years or sixty years. In this older age group options such as refractive lensectomy (clear lensectomy) may be a better option. Non-laser refractive surgery options are discussed in Chapter 13.

For younger people it is especially important to make sure that the eyeglass or contact lens prescription has been stable for at least one year and preferably for two years. Stability means that the correction should not have changed more that 0.25 to 0.50 diopters over the previous one to two years. For highly nearsighted people the refraction sometimes will not stabilize until they are twenty-five to thirty years old. If you have laser vision correction before your refraction is stable the eyes will naturally continue to progress and the nearsightedness or astigmatism will return. While it is possible to do an enhancement or touch-up at a later date, in most cases it is not advisable to do multiple enhancements.

For people approaching forty years old or who are in their forties, they must carefully consider the need for reading glasses. This age related loss of focus ability is called presbyopia. If you wear contact lenses for distance and are in your forties then you will find your vision for close work to be similar following laser vision correction. For those people who wear glasses or progressive lenses it is sometimes more difficult to determine how much your reading vision will be impacted.

Having laser vision correction is like pasting your contacts or distance glasses on permanently. There will be no progressive add to help with reading, and you will not have glasses or contacts to remove. If you have a full distance laser vision correction done on both eyes you will have to wear reading glasses starting sometime between about age forty years and forty-five years old. Reading glasses will be required for any close work including sewing, hobbies like model building, applying makeup, or any fine work within arms reach.

For those who wish to reduce dependence on readers, monovision can be done with contact lenses or with laser vision correction. Monovision is a compromise where one eye is corrected for full distance and the other eye is left with approximately 1.25 diopters nearsighted (more or less at the surgeon's discretion) for reading. The best way to find out if you are a good candidate for monovision is to do a trial for a few weeks with contact lenses. If you do not wear contacts, your eye doctor can show you what monovision will be like by setting up your correction in trial lenses which can be worn in the doctor's office.

There are many people who can not tolerate monovision due to an inability of their brain to adjust to the difference between eyes. Other people adjust easily but may still need to wear corrective lenses for distance activities such as night driving or for fine close work such as threading a needle. People with visually demanding hobbies like golf or tennis or occupations like driving may not be good candidates for monovision. If you are close to or in your forties you should talk to your eye care provider about what you can expect for close vision following laser vision correction and if you might be a candidate for monovision.

As people approach the late fifties and sixties they will have naturally progressed to where they will need a trifocal or progressive lens for their close and intermediate vision. Many people may have already switched to monovision

Chapter 3: Who is a Candidate for Laser Vision Correction?

with their contact lenses or will be wearing readers over their contacts. In this age group cataracts may begin to become more common. For these reasons, many surgeons will begin to prefer intraocular (inside the eye) surgeries like the implantable contact lens or clear lens replacement to reduce dependence on glasses or contact lenses. There are new intraocular lens implants that can be used for lens replacement that have the ability to focus to some degree at near. As these new intraocular lenses with the ability to focus become more widely used, it is possible that this might become the procedure of choice for the fifty-five and older group as it will also restore some of the close vision that was naturally lost with age.

There are some unique situations in which people over the age of sixty may benefit from laser vision correction. For example if unexpected nearsightedness or residual astigmatism occurs after cataract surgery a laser vision correction can be done to restore balance between eyes and improve uncorrected distance vision.

Occupation

Some occupations such as police, military, or pilots have specific rules about laser vision correction surgery. It is your responsibility to understand the rules and regulations regarding laser eye surgery and how it may affect your occupation. For example, pilots will likely be grounded for a period of time following laser eye surgery. Some occupations require color vision testing which is not a standard part of laser vision assessment. Most laser vision centers will test color vision if requested.

If you have a visually demanding career, be aware that the risk of a poor outcome from laser vision correction, although small, may include loss of ability to perform visually demanding tasks important for your occupation. Monovision is not recommended for those with visually demanding occupations.

Expectations

While most centers will not do any formal personality testing, it is well known that people with unrealistic expectations or who are very particular about their vision are more likely to be unhappy with the results of laser vision correction. You must be prepared to be patient with the healing, with recovery of night vision, and with the possible need for retreatment or enhancement. Approximately five to fifteen percent of people may need a second treatment for their best vision and may have to wait six months or longer before the correction is stable enough to proceed with a second treatment. Pre-existing mental health conditions such as untreated depression or anxiety may make it difficult for you to adjust if you have a complication from laser vision correction surgery.

People who are very sensitive to their vision should think carefully about undertaking a laser vision correction. While most people have excellent results, it is not possible to do repeat surgeries for very fine adjustments, and it is not advisable to do multiple retreatments. Glasses and contacts can be adjusted whenever you wish even if the change is quite small. If you require frequent small adjustments of your corrective lenses you may not be a good candidate for laser vision correction.

If you are very conservative and uncomfortable taking even a small risk, laser vision correction may not be a good option for you. Although the risk is low, if you are one of the rare people to suffer a permanent reduction in vision as a result of laser vision correction you must be prepared to cope with an unfortunate outcome.

Hobbies

Those with visually demanding hobbies such as golf or tennis may find they are not satisfied until the long term healing is completed over a number of weeks to months. It is possible that vision may not be as sharp after laser

Chapter 3: Who is a Candidate for Laser Vision Correction?

vision correction under low lighting conditions such as a cloudy day or at dusk on a permanent basis. Monovision is not recommended for people with visually demanding hobbies.

Hobbies or sports that are high risk for eye injury include basketball, hockey, kick-boxing, and other sports. Safety glasses are always recommended for any sports or activities where eye injury may occur even if you do not undergo surgery. Those considering laser vision correction may wish to consider a no-flap procedure to eliminate the risk of flap shift from trauma weeks, months, or years after surgery.

If you are mildly to moderately nearsighted and have hobbies which involve close work such as music, sewing, or model building you will lose your ability to do these close tasks without glasses if you are over the age of forty and have both eyes corrected fully for distance. Be sure to discuss how surgery may affect your hobbies with your surgeon prior to considering laser vision correction.

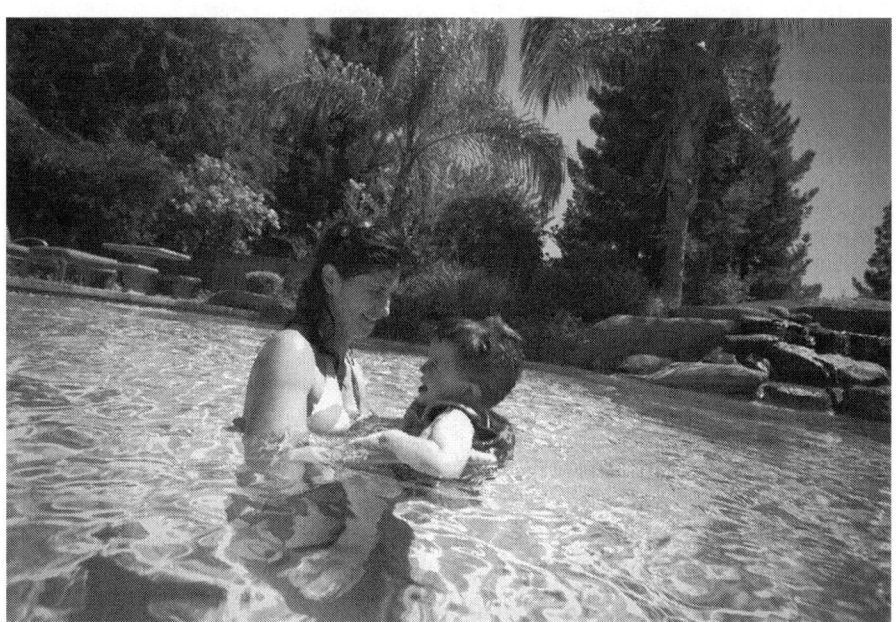

Nearsightedness (Myopia)

The technical term for nearsightedness is myopia. Please refer to Chapter 2 for an in depth discussion of myopia. For the nearsighted eye the minimum correction for some surgeons for laser vision correction is −1.00 diopter. For the very low corrections it may not be worth the risk of performing laser vision correction since many people with low corrections only wear their glasses occasionally and already enjoy a variety of activities without glasses.

Laser vision correction in most cases can be done for nearsighted corrections up to −10.00 diopters. If the cornea has adequate thickness, higher corrections may be considered. As the correction becomes higher the corneal thickness becomes more important. There are guidelines that are used to determine if you are a candidate for a deeper flap based procedure such as LASIK or Intra-LASIK or if a surface procedure such as PRK or Epi-LASIK may be a better choice (the surface treatments will always leave more corneal tissue untouched, so if you qualify for a flap based procedure you will qualify for the surface treatments as well). There may be a few nearsighted people with corrections higher than -10.00 diopters that may qualify for laser vision correction, and there may be a few people with very thin corneas and corrections lower than −10.00 who may not be good candidates for laser vision corrections.

Farsightedness (Hyperopia)

For the farsighted person, also known as hyperopic, the guidelines for laser vision corrected will usually include a range of about +1.00 to +3.50. There are some surgeons who may treat higher hyperopia. Farsightedness is discussed in detail in Chapter 2. Farsighted people are able to compensate for their farsightedness by using their natural focusing ability. Since the natural focusing ability weakens

Chapter 3: Who is a Candidate for Laser Vision Correction?

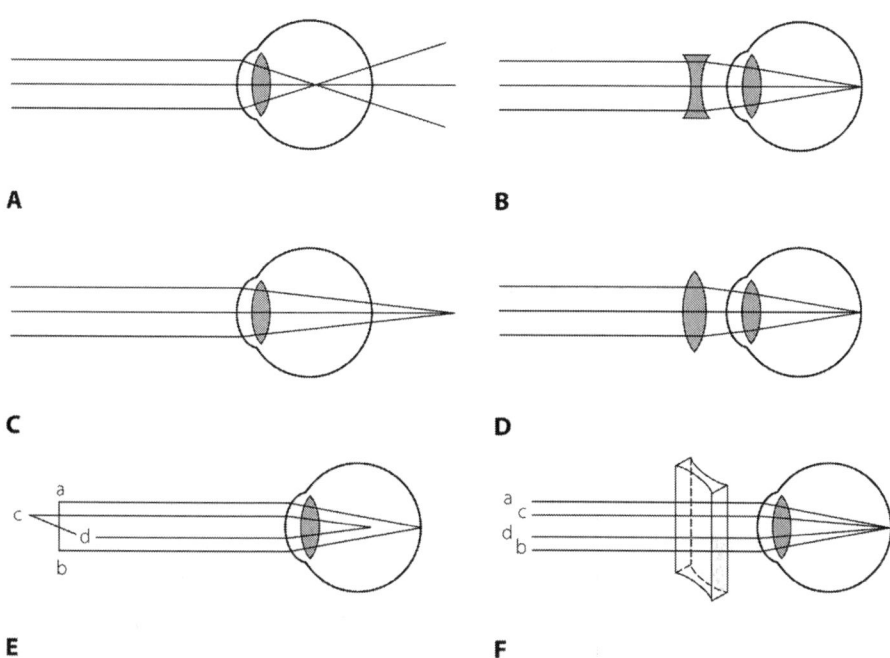

Concave lenses correct for nearsightedness, convex lenses for farsightedness, and toric lenses for astigmatism. The excimer laser reshapes the cornea to reduce or eliminate the need for corrective lenses. © 2009 American Academy of Ophthalmology

with age, many farsighted people will first need reading glasses in their twenties or thirties and may not need distance glasses until they are closer to forty or fifty.

If you are farsighted it is especially important to have an eyeglass check with the eyes dilated, called a cycloplegic or "wet" refraction, to uncover the true amount of farsightedness present. The dilating drops make the pupil large and also temporarily relax the focusing muscle in the eye. The cycloplegic or "wet" refraction is the only way to determine the full amount of farsightedness present.

Astigmatism

Astigmatism up to approximately 4.50 diopters and sometimes higher can be treated with laser vision correction along with any nearsightedness or farsightedness that is present. Chapter 2 includes a detailed description of astigmatism. Astigmatism in most cases means that the surface of the cornea is shaped like a barrel or a football with two different curvatures at ninety degrees to each other from steepest to flattest. Laser vision correction for astigmatism reshapes the corneal surface from a football shape to a basketball shape or sphere.

Very high astigmatism, changing astigmatism, or irregular astigmatism (where the steepest and flattest curvatures are less than ninety degrees apart) can indicate the presence of a corneal disorder such as keratoconus or pellucid dystrophy. Corneal disorders such as these can lead to corneal instability (ectasia) and a changing correction with or without laser vision correction. These types of corneal conditions are absolute contraindications to laser refractive surgery and will usually be detected with corneal mapping.

Corneal Thickness

Laser vision correction should be approached cautiously for people with corneas thinner than 500 microns. There is no established minimum at this time for the residual thickness that should be left after surface treatments such as PRK or Epi-LASIK and unpublished guidelines range from 350 to 440 microns for final corneal thickness which includes the epithelium which is 40 to 50 microns thick.

For flap based treatments such as LASIK and Intra-LASIK the recommended amount of cornea that should remain untouched is 250 to 300 microns which is theoretically necessary to provide enough structural integrity to the cornea. Although the flap is not removed, once it is created it may not contribute to the corneal strength. A good analogy is to compare the flap to the cables on the Golden Gate Bridge. If you cut some of the bridge cables, they will still be hanging there but will no longer be holding the bridge up. Since different microkeratomes and femtosecond lasers

Chapter 3: Who is a Candidate for Laser Vision Correction?

will create different flap thicknesses, your suitability for these procedures will be determined at the assessment based on your individual correction and corneal thickness.

If a cornea is thinned too far it may present a risk for corneal instability called ectasia. Ectasia is rare but very hard to treat. When the cornea is thinned too far it is like a weak spot in a tire. The thinner areas tend to bulge out and create irregular astigmatism. There are other risk factors for ectasia including abnormal corneal maps, unstable prescription, and family history of keratoconus. Additional laser surgery can not be done in these cases and specialized contact lenses, corneal cross-linking surgery, or corneal transplant may be required.

Corneal Mapping

Corneal mapping is an essential part of the laser vision correction assessment. Corneal mapping is done to check for corneal conditions such as keratoconus or pellucid dystrophy. Your surgeon will determine your candidacy for laser vision correction from the corneal maps as well as the other measurements taken during your assessment.

Contact lenses will warp the corneal surface and for that reason you will be required to leave your contact lenses out for a period of time prior to corneal mapping and prior to laser vision correction. For wavefront measurements to be used in custom wavefront laser vision correction there may be a longer period of time that you will have to be out of contact lenses since these measurements will be entered into the laser to customize your correction. It is to your benefit to leave the contact lenses out for the requested time period in order for the measurements to be as accurate as possible.

Dry eye can also affect the mapping patterns. If the maps show irregularity in a dry eye or in a situation where contacts have been worn recently, the maps may need to be repeated for accuracy after a longer period out of

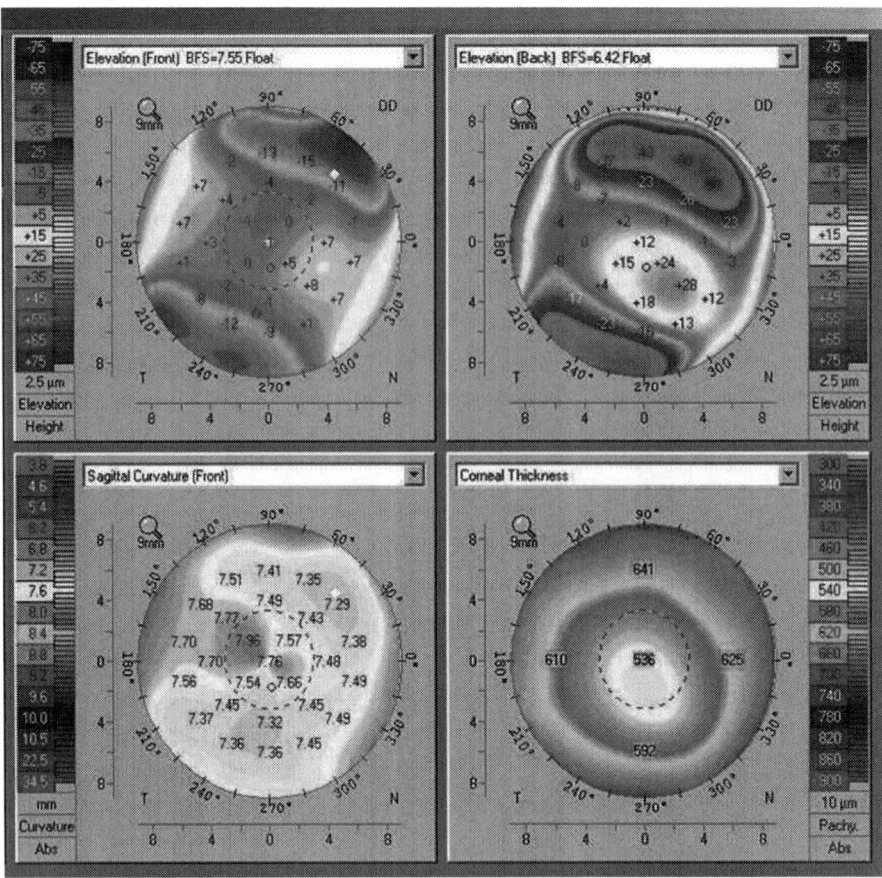

Corneal mapping measures the shape of the cornea. © 2009 American Academy of Ophthalmology

contact lenses. You may also be asked to use artificial tears on a regular schedule for a few days to a week before repeat mapping.

Past History of Eye Disease

There are many types of eye disease that may impact your suitability for laser vision correction. The list below contains a few of the more common conditions.

Chapter 3: Who is a Candidate for Laser Vision Correction?

Eye diseases that may affect candidacy for surgery:

Corneal dystrophy:	keratoconus and pellucid dystrophy are contraindications.
Cataracts:	cataract surgery or lens replacement may be a better option.
Retinal detachment:	treated detachments may limit vision after surgery.
Glaucoma:	eye drops used for glaucoma treatment may affect healing.
Dry eye:	severe dry eye may be a contraindication for surgery.
Lid disorders:	may pose a risk for complications.
Prior history of ocular herpes:	may disqualify you for surgery.
Double vision:	surgery may worsen a pre-existing condition.
Iritis:	inflammation inside the eye may pose a risk for abnormal healing.

Your surgeon should discuss your eye health with you prior to surgery, identify eye diseases that need treatment, identify eye disease that may put you at higher risk for complications of laser vision correction, and identify eye diseases which will disqualify you for laser vision correction.

Past history of keratoconus or pellucid dystrophy will disqualify you for laser vision correction. If you have cataracts you may be a better candidate for an intraocular procedure such as clear lens replacement or implantable contact lenses.

Other eye diseases such as retinal detachment, glaucoma, diabetic retinopathy, or macular degeneration may impact what you can expect from laser vision correction but do not automatically disqualify you from laser vision correction. Dry eye is a common condition that may be worsened with laser vision correction. Severe dry eye may disqualify you from laser vision correction. If you have a history of double vision or wandering eye, laser vision correction may be a risk for worsening of the pre-existing eye muscle imbalance. Previous history of ocular herpes simplex (HSV) or ocular herpes zoster which is also known as shingles may disqualify you for surgery.

Your surgeon will determine based on your own individual eye history and eye examination how pre-existing eye conditions might affect your results from laser vision correction. Specialized testing such as visual field analysis might be required before laser vision correction. You should be sure to mention all previous eye diseases, prior eye surgeries, or previous injuries at the assessment and ask if you are at higher risk for complications of laser vision correction if you have any pre-existing conditions.

Family History of Eye Disease

If you have a family history of keratoconus or pellucid dystrophy you may be at risk for ectasia (corneal instability) following laser vision correction. Other hereditary eye diseases may not disqualify you for laser vision correction but are important for your eye doctor to know about in order to provide the best care and recommendations for your overall eye health. Conditions such as glaucoma, retinal detachment, and macular degeneration can run in families.

Medical History

It is important to list all pre-existing medical conditions and medications including over the counter or herbal medications on your history form. In particular any active auto-immune disorder such as rheumatoid arthritis or

Chapter 3: Who is a Candidate for Laser Vision Correction?

systemic lupus may disqualify you for laser vision correction. Chronic conditions such as diabetes are not necessarily a contraindication for surgery however the blood sugar levels and eyeglass prescription should be stable.

Medical disorders that affect candidacy for laser vision correction:

Autoimmune disease:	disorders such as lupus and rheumatoid arthritis may put you at risk for serious complications following laser vision correction.
Diabetes:	people with stable blood sugars without retinopathy may qualify.
Pregnancy:	hormonal changes with pregnancy and breast feeding can cause refractive instability and can affect healing after surgery.

Your surgeon should discuss any concerns relating to your medical history prior to recommending laser vision correction.

Eye Examination

The assessment will include a dilated eye examination along with the specialized testing described earlier. The examining doctor will look at all the structures including the tear film, cornea, iris, lens, vitreous, optic nerve, and retina. For more information on basic anatomy refer to Chapter 7. Your prescription will be measured and compared to your previous correction to assess stability. In some cases the surgeon may request more information from previous eye examinations.

Pre-operative assessment should include these measurements:

Vision with glasses:	you will be advised to leave contacts out for 2 to 7 days prior to the assessment.
Corneal mapping:	this test can detect disorders such as keratoconus
Wavefront mapping:	for systems that have the capacity to do customized wavefront treatments a specialized map is used to measure aberrations.
Pupil size:	pupils will be assessed in dim and room light.
Manifest refraction:	eyeglass check done without dilating drops.
Cycloplegic refraction:	eyeglass check done after relaxing the focusing muscle with dilating drops.
Keratometry:	measurement of the corneal curvature.
Pachymetry:	measurement of corneal thickness.
Slit lamp examination:	microscopic examination of the eye.
Indirect ophthalmoscopy:	examination of the peripheral retina.

Following the examination, corneal mapping, and corneal thickness measurements your surgeon will determine if you qualify for laser vision correction and what procedure is recommended. If any abnormalities are found on the eye examination your surgeon may require additional testing before allowing you to undergo laser vision correction.

Summary

In most cases the laser center staff will have a list of questions to ask when you make your assessment appointment. In some cases a person might be ruled out based on this initial questioning without undergoing a complete assessment. For example, someone with active rheumatoid arthritis or a family history of keratoconus would not be a candidate for laser vision correction. Although it is disappointing if you are disqualified, it is important to give all the information to the laser center staff and surgeon in order to make a well informed and safe decision regarding your suitability for laser vision correction.

CHAPTER 4: HOW TO CHOOSE A SURGEON

When considering laser vision correction, there are a number of things for the potential candidate to consider including price, location, procedure type, and surgeon. Surgeons who perform laser vision correction in the United States and Canada are required to have certain qualifications including a medical license. In spite of these requirements, there may be important differences between surgeons that you may wish to consider when deciding where to have laser vision correction.

Surgeon Qualifications

Your surgeon will be an ophthalmologist. An ophthalmologist is a medical doctor (MD) or Doctor of Osteopathy (DO) with a four year general medical degree plus additional years of training in an ophthalmology residency. Residency is when an ophthalmologist, also sometimes called an Eye MD, learns to take care of general eye disorders, learns general eye surgery techniques, and in some cases will take training in specific surgery such as PRK, Intra-LASIK, LASIK, or Epi-LASIK.

Basic Surgeon Qualifications:

Education: minimum includes MD or DO plus an ophthalmology residency.

Licensure: state or provincial licenses are required for practice.

Board certification: most North American surgeons will be board certified through the American Board of Ophthalmology or the Royal College of Physicians and Surgeons of Canada.

Fellowship: some surgeons will have additional training in refractive surgery or corneal disorders.

Training: each laser system and device requires specialized training.

Experience: you should feel free to ask how many cases your surgeon has done.

Accreditation: hospitals and outpatient surgery centers usually are required by state or provincial law to accredit surgeons who operate in the facility.

Some surgeons will do an additional year or two of training following medical school and ophthalmology residency. This additional training is called a fellowship. Not all laser vision correction surgeons will have fellowship training. Most often if a laser vision correction surgeon has a fellowship it will be in corneal disease or in refractive (laser vision correction) surgery.

Chapter 4: How to Choose a Surgeon

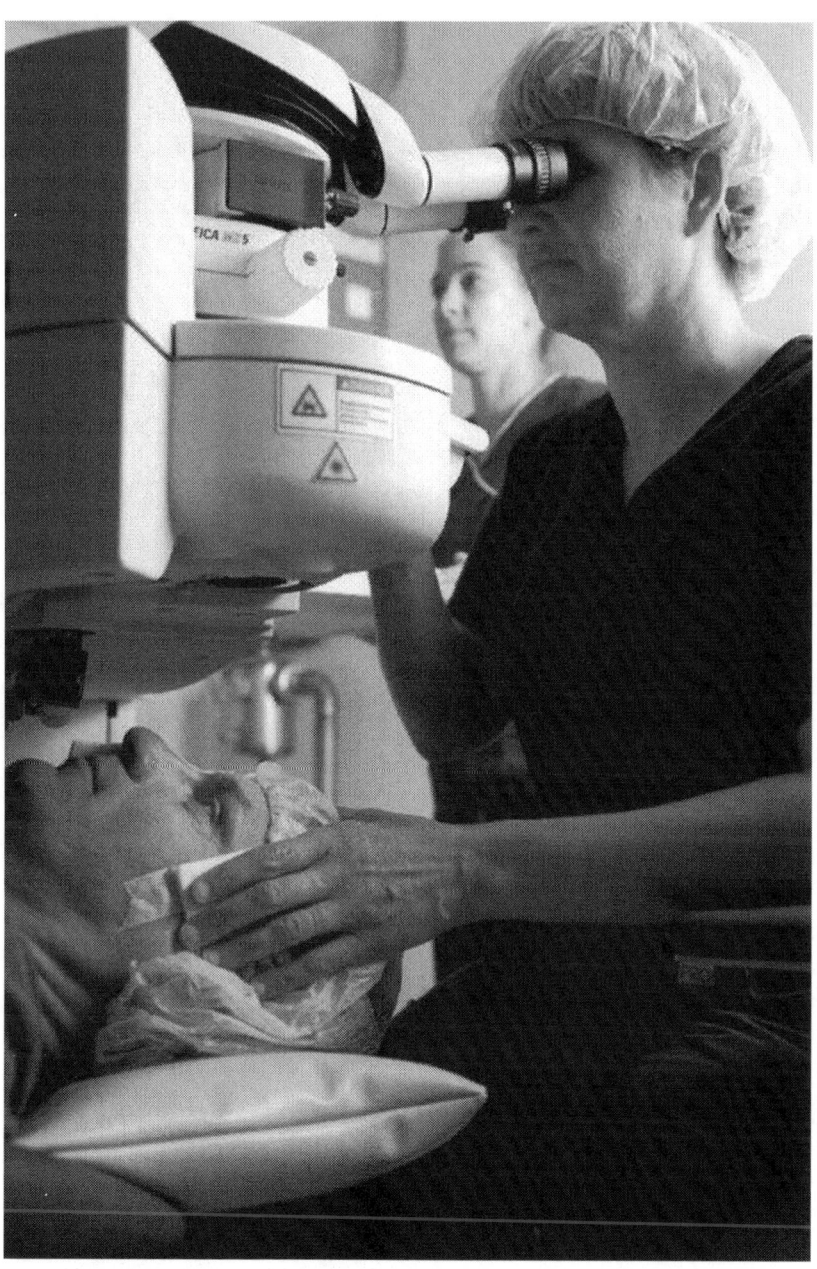

Photo by Dave Best.

Ophthalmologists, Eye MDs, differ from optometrists who are required to complete a doctorate of optometry but do not do a residency. Optometrists are designated by "OD" and do not do eye surgery. Optometrists are well qualified to do general eye care and treat a number of eye diseases. Optometrists will refer to ophthalmologists where more complex care or surgery is required. At some laser vision centers an optometrist will complete your assessment and provide post-operative care. In some cases, your usual optometrist will resume care as early as one week following your laser vision correction procedure.

Most North American laser vision correction surgeons will be board certified by the American Board of Ophthalmology or by the Royal College of Physicians and Surgeons of Canada. These board certifications are indicated by "Diplomate ABO" or "FRCSC" following the surgeon's name. Board certification is an important credential because it demonstrates that your laser vision correction surgeon has completed comprehensive training in eye care, treatment of eye diseases, and eye surgery. Most laser vision correction surgeons will have this information available on their website or in a bio that will be available in the laser vision center.

Chapter 4: How to Choose a Surgeon

What do all those letters behind the doctor's name mean?

MD: Medical Doctor degree signifies a four year medical degree.

OD: Doctor of Optometry degree signifies a four year optometry degree.

DO: Doctor of Osteopathy degree signifies a four year osteopathic degree.

FRCSC: Fellow of the Royal College of Physicians and Surgeons of Canada designation signifies board certification in Canada.

Diplomate ABO: Diplomate of the American Board of Ophthalmology designation signifies board certification in the United States.

MS: Masters degree in Science degree is a post undergraduate university degree which is usually completed in two years.

Ph.D.: Doctorate of Philosophy degree is a post undergraduate university degree which takes a variable amount of time to complete depending on the field.

B.S.: Bachelor of Science degree signifies a four year undergraduate university degree

B.A.: Bachelor of Arts degree signifies a four year undergraduate university degree

Surgeon Experience

Most established laser vision correction surgeons will have the basic qualifications described above, but experience will vary. As with any activity experience will be of benefit to both patient and surgeon. An experienced surgeon may be able to detect conditions before surgery that might present a higher risk for laser vision correction. Experience also helps in cases where there is a complication at the time of the procedure or following the procedure.

Studies have shown that complication rates decline with surgeon experience. Unfortunately there is no magic number of cases to use as a deciding point when choosing a surgeon. Some people wish to go with a surgeon that has done at least 100 laser vision correction surgeries and others may wish to choose a surgeon who has done over 1000 surgeries. There are some advertisements that mention specific numbers of surgeries done. Be sure to find out how many of these were laser vision correction procedures and more specifically how many cases have been done of the specific type that you are considering.

There is some debate about what kind of experience a surgeon should have. Some feel that a laser vision correction surgeon should have performed a number of different types of corrective surgeries and others feel it is more important that the surgeon is an expert in the particular procedure they are choosing. Some surgeons will specialize in the procedure that they feel offers the best outcomes and highest level of safety in their hands. There are some centers that offer only Epi-LASIK or PRK and other centers that rarely do anything other than LASIK. The reasons for these differences include surgeon experience, surgeon preference, philosophies of care, and advances in technology. You should feel free to discuss with your surgeon their reasons for recommending a particular procedure.

It is important for you to know who will be doing your surgery. If you undergo an assessment with a larger center with multiple surgeons, you may not meet your surgeon until

Chapter 4: How to Choose a Surgeon

the day of the laser vision correction procedure. Some centers will have ophthalmologists in training, residents or fellows, observe or participate in your surgical care. In general you will be given the choice as to whether to book with an ophthalmologist in training. In these cases the ophthalmologist in training may be directly supervised by a more senior ophthalmologist. You may choose to request a senior surgeon, or if you are comfortable with the ophthalmologist in residency or fellowship training you may choose that surgeon.

Who is a surgeon in training?

Medical student:	a student who is currently undertaking a four year medical degree. Often will observe and may do simple examinations.
Resident in ophthalmology:	an MD or DO who is undertaking an additional four to five years of training to specialize in ophthalmology. A resident may be participating in all or part of a surgical case.
Fellow:	an MD or DO who has completed a residency in ophthalmology and is undertaking sub-specialty training such as refractive surgery or cornea. Fellows will usually be doing surgeries with or without supervision.

Surgeon Availability

There is usually a higher cost for laser vision correction at centers where the surgeon spends more time with the potential candidate before and after surgery. The reason for this is simple economics. The ophthalmic surgeon is the engine of any ophthalmology practice. Their work needs to cover all of the costs associated with running a laser vision center. This overhead is substantial and includes the cost of sophisticated lasers, corneal mapping and other specialized devices, personnel, advertising, rent, utilities, supplies, and many other items that are critical to a well run center. There is a cost versus volume relationship in laser vision correction pricing. The lower the price of the procedure, the more surgeries have to be done per day or per week.

There are many very well qualified high volume ophthalmic surgeons working at low cost centers. If you choose to go with these centers you will most likely have technical staff doing the majority of your assessment and your post-operative care, but you may not see the surgeon at the pre- and post-operative visits. In some cases the surgeon may travel from another state or province for the day of surgery. You will in most cases have a short meeting with the surgeon just prior to your procedure. If you are planning to have your laser vision correction at a high volume center, be sure to ask who is available for after hours care.

If it is important to you to have a more lengthy consultation with your laser vision correction surgeon you will likely pay a higher price than you will at the higher volume centers. The disadvantage of a lower volume center is usually a higher price. The advantages include a more in depth discussion with your surgeon prior to choosing to undergo laser vision correction and a more in depth discussion with your surgeon of why a particular procedure is recommended. In some smaller centers the surgeon will also provide your post-operative care. This will allow you to ask questions or raise concerns directly with your surgeon at any of the post-procedure visits rather than having to schedule additional appointments to meet with your surgeon.

No matter which choice you make, high volume/low cost or lower volume/higher cost, be sure to understand the choice you are making by asking questions before your laser vision correction surgery.

Chapter 4: How to Choose a Surgeon

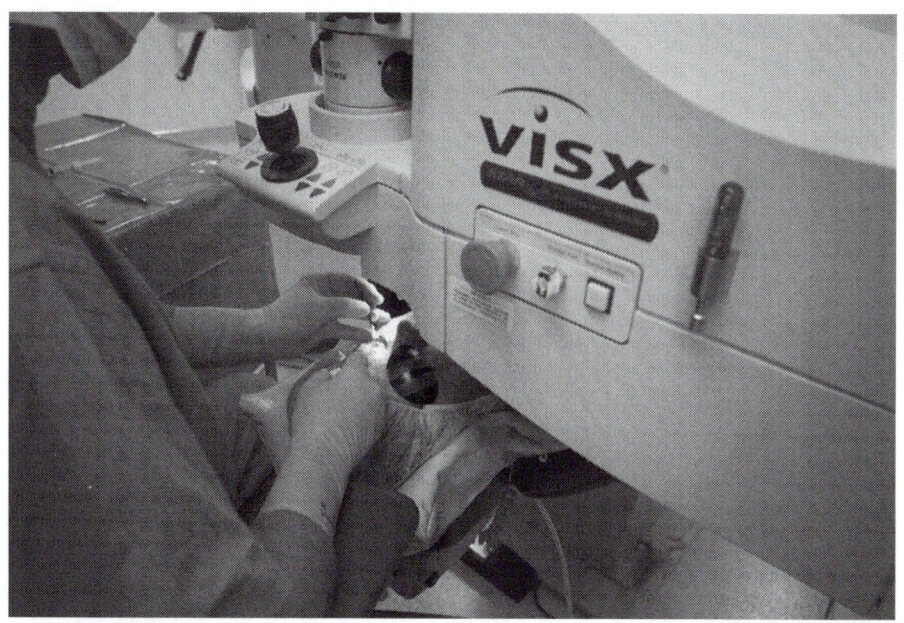

Surgeon Approachability

An experienced surgeon should welcome any questions you have and should easily admit when they do not know the answer to a question. There are a staggering amount of details that a surgeon may be considering when making recommendations. Add to that an ever changing technologic landscape including software and hardware updates and it is likely that if you ask enough questions you will be likely to ask something that even the surgeon may have to look up. A good surgeon may tell you they do not know the answer but will research it.

In spite of advancing technology it is still not possible to foresee all risks and complications. You should feel free to ask as many questions as you need to in order to feel comfortable with your choice of whether to proceed with laser vision correction and with the specific procedure you may be considering.

Surgeon Equipment

There have been significant changes in technology since Dr. Margueritte MacDonald performed the first PRK in the U.S. in 1988. Each laser center will have a unique set of instruments including different laser types with may be capable of different types of laser vision correction techniques. The major differences will include flap making devices for LASIK or Intra-LASIK, devices to remove the epithelium for Epi-LASIK, and laser types for doing standard or custom wavefront laser correction. Custom wavefront treatments can be done with PRK, Epi-LASIK, LASIK, or Intra-LASIK.

FDA approved excimer lasers at this time:

MEL 80 Excimer:	Carl Zeiss, Inc.
Wavelight Allegretto Wave Excimer:	Alcon Laboratories, Inc.
Technolas 217A Excimer:	Technolas GMBH Perfect Vision
VISX Excimer:	AMO
Laserscan LSX excimer:	Lasersight Technologies Inc
Bausch & Lomb Keracor 116 Excimer:	Technolas GMBH Perfect Vision
EC-5000 Excimer:	Nidek Inc.
LADARVISION Excimer:	Alcon Laboratories Inc.
Kremer Laser Systems:	Lasersight Technologies Inc.

Excimer lasers will generally fall into one of three categories – scanning spot, scanning slit, or broad beam lasers. This subject will be covered in more detail in Chapter 12. Some lasers have the capability to do a true wavefront correction and others may use a more standard format. You should familiarize yourself with the laser in use at the center where you are considering having laser vision correction.

There is considerable debate regarding flap or no-flap procedures as well as what is called Sub-Bowmans Keratomeliusis (SBK) and Intra-LASIK. SBK is a newer thin flap LASIK technique. If you plan to undergo a procedure in which a flap is created there are microkeratomes which can create a very thin flap which some experts feel is as good as the flap created by the femtosecond laser in Intra-LASIK. There are other experts who feel strongly that the no-flap procedures of PRK and Epi-LASIK provide equally good long term outcomes with a better level of safety. This group of experts believes that the longer recovery in the first weeks after the procedure is a worthwhile investment of time in return for lower risk. A detailed description of these procedures and the current technology available can be found in Part II.

Whether you are interested in researching the details of the wide array of technology available for laser vision correction or you choose to rely on the advice of your surgeon, you may wish to learn the basics of what is available in order to understand the choice you are making for laser vision correction.

Surgeon Location

There may be reasons why you may be looking at traveling to another location for surgery. Consider your options carefully in this regard. If you are traveling to another city or country to save money, be aware that while most surgeons will make every effort to remedy a complication you will have to travel back to that location to receive care. If you have surgery in one location and seek care for a complication closer to home, it is likely to cost as much as the original surgery.

Usually there are one or more eye examinations needed within the first few days of a laser vision correction surgery. In an uncomplicated case your next visit will be anywhere from one week to one month. Depending on the type of laser vision correction is done there may be a need for monthly visits for a few months while healing is taking place.

Co-management

In cases where the surgery center is located far away, some surgeons are agreeable to co-managing with another ophthalmologist or optometrist. For this type of arrangement to work there must be good communication between providers. Both the surgeon the eye care provider who will be doing follow up care must agree in advance in order for co-management to be effective. If there is a late complication the follow-up provider must be able to communicate with the surgeon and arrange additional visits or treatments with the surgeon if necessary. This arrangement works well for those who may live in more rural areas where they may have to travel into a metropolitan center to access laser vision correction.

Co-management

Co-management:	describes an arrangement between the surgery center and another eye care provider such as an optometrist.
Communication:	for co-management arrangements to work there must be excellent communication between the surgeon and the co-manager.
Benefit:	for some people co-management is a great option due to geographic reasons, if their usual provider has better hours, or if they wish to continue care with a trusted provider.

Surgery Center Staff

You will spend more time with the surgery center staff than you will with your surgeon. From the receptionist or secretary who will book your appointments to the technical staff who will do your pre-testing and operating room staff who will make sure you are comfortable during your procedure, you should pay attention to the surgery center staff. Many centers also have counselors who will provide pre-operative information.

During the assessment you will be likely to meet many of the staff who you will be interacting with if you choose to book surgery. While there are many factors that will influence your decision about whether or where to have laser vision correction, be sure to make note of the surgery center staff when making your choice. Many staff members of laser vision correction centers have had refractive surgery themselves and can be good resources for information.

The types of staff that will participate in your care may include a certified ophthalmic assistant (COA), certified ophthalmic technician (COT), or certified ophthalmic medical technologist (COMT). More information on these designations can be found in Chapter 1.

Referral to a Surgeon

It can be helpful to ask your medical doctor or optometrist for a referral to a laser vision correction surgeon they trust. Most doctors will only refer to surgeons that have provided good care in the past. It would be unlikely that a reputable doctor would continue to refer to a laser vision correction surgeon who did not provide good results.

Word of Mouth

Another way to find a laser vision correction surgeon is to speak to family and friends. You will want to think carefully about choosing a surgeon or laser center that has had a

Laser Vision Correction

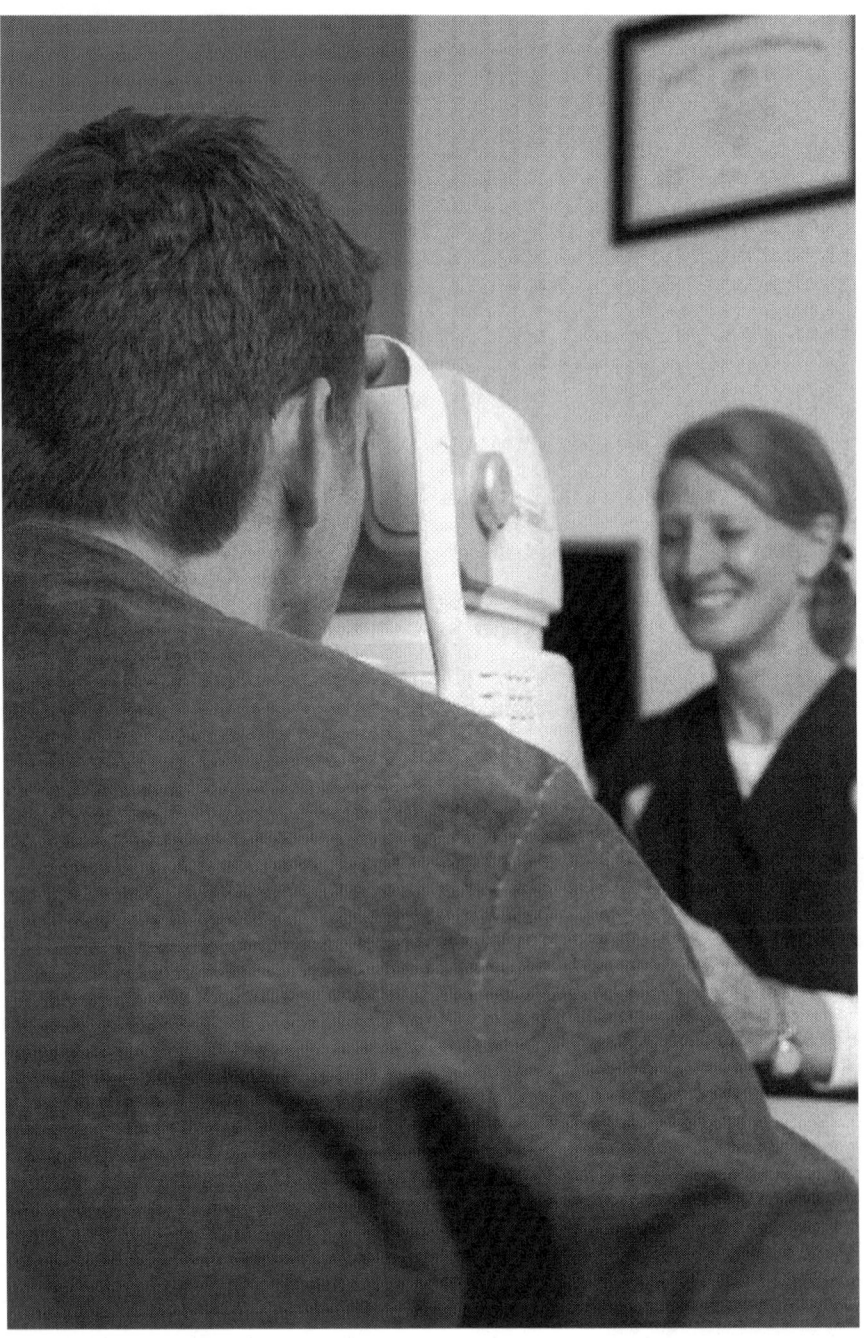

Photo by Dave Best.

Chapter 4: How to Choose a Surgeon

large volume of complaints, but keep in mind that any surgeon who has performed hundreds or thousands of surgeries is likely to have had some complications in their career. My mentor, a phenomenal refractive surgeon Dr. Howard Gimbel, feels the mark of a good surgeon is not whether or not there have been any complications but how the surgeon managed those complications. Any surgeon who says they have never had a complication has probably not done a lot of cases. So a bad outcome does not necessarily mean the surgeon was at fault.

When you speak to family and friends you may learn about the surgeon's bedside manner and about the staff at the laser center. In some cases some people who have had complications of laser vision correction may still recommend their surgeon due to the quality care they received. If there are many happy patrons of a particular center then it is likely that the staff and surgeon are well qualified.

Websites

Surgery Center websites will often contain pages describing the credentials of the surgeon or surgeons at a particular laser vision correction center. These websites may also provide information about the types of procedures performed, numbers of procedures performed, and technology available at the center. A list of reliable websites for general laser vision correction information can be found in Chapter 1.

Second Opinions

Although a full laser vision correction assessment can take two to three hours to complete, it may be worthwhile to have more than one assessment at different centers. This allows you to meet the staff and at small centers may allow you to meet with the surgeon as well prior to booking laser vision correction. You will be able to get an individualized quote as well as information on what the pricing includes.

In this way you can compare prices and services at more than one center.

It is possible that you may be given different recommendations at different centers. The reasons for this include differences between surgeon practice, and differences between surgeon experience. For example, a surgeon who may have done numerous procedures with a specific laser may be more comfortable with more complex or higher corrections.

Each laser has different capabilities and so a surgeon with access to a specific laser may have recommendations that may differ from one who uses a different laser. The same is true of flap versus no-flap recommendations. Surgeon experience may play a role in recommendations. In many cases you may qualify for more than one procedure. If this is the case you will need to weigh the risks and benefits of each procedure (and the option of no surgery) and make your decision accordingly.

Summary

There are a number of things to consider when choosing a surgeon for laser vision correction. You should feel as comfortable with your choice of surgeon as you are with your choice of which procedure to have. Your surgeon should welcome any questions you may have about laser vision correction.

CHAPTER 5: HOW TO CHOOSE BETWEEN PRK, EPI-LASIK, LASIK, OR INTRA-LASIK

The large volume of advertisements, news stories, and scientific publications about laser vision correction can be overwhelming and confusing. In many cases there are competing articles and advertisements each claiming that their technique is the best and latest available to consumers.

Even the scientific journals produce conflicting reports and experts continuously debate the pros and cons of the various laser vision correction surgeries at annual meetings such as the Annual Meeting of the Academy of Ophthalmology and the Annual Meeting of the American Society of Cataract and Refractive Surgeons. Similar meetings and similar debates occur in Europe, Asia, and across the world.

For the expert and consumer alike the amount of information is overwhelming to try to understand. It can be helpful to simplify the choices by considering what things

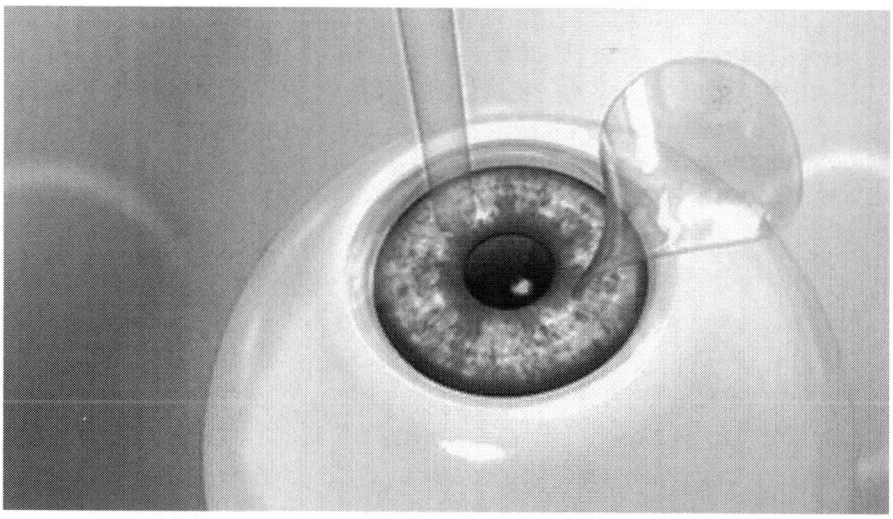

LASIK and Intralasik both involve the creation of a corneal flap that is lifted with the laser treatment applied to the underlying bed. PRK and Epi-LASIK are surface no flap treatments which reshape the outermost part of the cornea.

are the same between procedures and what things are different. Each of these techniques will be discussed in more detail in Part II of this book.

Similarities Between PRK, Epi-LASIK, LASIK, and Intra-LASIK

The following things are the same regardless of the type of laser vision correction procedure you choose:

Similarities Between All Laser Vision Surgeries

- You will have to undergo an assessment as described in Chapter 3 to determine if you qualify for laser vision correction.
- There is some risk to any of the laser vision correction procedures. No technique is risk free.
- There is a chance you will need a retreatment for your best vision.
- The most common side effects of all of the laser vision correction techniques are dry eye and rarely glare or halo with night vision.
- The goal of all laser vision correction procedures is to reduce your dependence on glasses. None of the techniques will result in better vision than you have with your most up to date glasses or contact lenses.
- If you are forty to forty-five or older you will need reading glasses for close work unless you choose monovision as discussed in Chapters 2 and 3.
- PRK, Epi-LASIK, LASIK, and Intra-LASIK all have excellent long term results. To date there have been no large scale studies to prove that the visual outcomes are better with any one of these laser vision correction techniques.
- Custom wavefront or other types of customized laser vision correction can be done with any of these techniques.

Chapter 5: How to Choose Between PRK, Epi-LASIK, LASIK, or Intra-LASIK

Differences: Flap (LASIK and Intra-LASIK) Versus No-Flap (PRK and Epi-LASIK)

As mentioned above, the long term outcomes of any of these procedures are equally good. The main difference between a flap based procedure and a no-flap surface treatment is that creating a flap carries a higher level of risk and gives more rapid recovery of vision in the first few days following surgery.

The risk of complications with flap creation is low, but it is possible that irregularities in the flap such as a buttonhole or partial flap may occur at the time of surgery. With no-flap techniques there is no flap to become involved in that type of intra-operative complication so the risk is lower. The flap may also be damaged or shifted months or years after surgery. This is very uncommon and in most cases the flap can be replaced and smoothed back into position with additional surgery.

There are a number of additional possible complications that are uncommon but can occur following a flap based procedure. I have co-authored the book "LASIK Complications" which has been translated into Spanish and Japanese and has gone into three editions. There is no book called PRK Complications. The reason is that there are fewer complications that can occur with no-flap treatments. While the risk of the no-flap procedures is not zero, it is lower because there is no flap that can become involved in these types of complications.

The reason the flap based procedures are so much more popular is due to the more rapid recovery of vision and earlier return to work. Most people are back to work within one to two days, although the night vision may take longer to recover. With no-flap procedures approximately one week is required to recover useful vision and the vision may sharpen up over a few weeks to a month following surgery. Most people undergoing laser vision correction with a no-flap technique will plan to take about a week off of work and may need assistance with young children or other duties for the first three days following surgery.

The other reason that flap based procedures became quickly popular when introduced in the 1990s has to do with the older excimer laser technology and the past tendency for the formation of scarring and haze with PRK. Due to advancements in laser technology, medications, and surgical techniques the risk of visually significant haze is very low now.

The most feared complication of the flap based procedures is corneal instability called ectasia. Risk factors for ectasia are touched on in Chapters 2 and 3, and ectasia will be discussed in more detail in Chapters 10 and 11. Ectasia has been reported following PRK but is much more common with LASIK. Intra-LASIK lasers and newer SBK (sub-Bowmans keratomeleusis) microkeratomes create very thin flaps which are thought to reduce the risk of ectasia. Thin flap techniques are very new and the prevalence of ectasia with thin flaps may not be known for several years as this condition can develop any time from immediately post-operatively to several years following surgery.

There is a significant amount of discussion recently about the risk factors for ectasia and the corneal biomechanics of creating a corneal flap. Some risk factors have been identified but there are some cases of ectasia in which no risk factors were apparent. Risk factors may include corneal mapping abnormalities, thin corneas, and family history of keratoconus.

Ectasia can not be corrected by further laser vision correction and requires treatment with customized contact lenses or in severe cases with corneal transplant. There are some surgeons who will only perform no-flap procedures due to this risk of ectasia, some are turning to thin flap procedures to reduce the risk, and others feel the risk of ectasia is so low that it is reasonable to give people a choice of procedures.

Differences Between Surgeries

PRK & Epi-LASIK: no flap treatments with laser applied to corneal surface after surface epithelial cells are removed.

Chapter 5: How to Choose Between PRK, Epi-LASIK, LASIK, or Intra-LASIK

LASIK & Intra-LASIK: flap is created and the laser is applied to the interior corneal bed under the flap.

PRK: surface epithelial cells are removed using a brush or by using a dilute alcohol solution to soften the cells followed by manual removal.

Epi-LASIK: surface cells are removed using an epikeratome device with an epithelial separator which uses a suction ring to stabilize the eye.

LASIK: the flap is made using a microkeratome device with an oscillating blade; a suction ring is used to stabilize the eye.

Intra-LASIK: a femtosecond laser is used to create a corneal flap using a suction ring to stabilize the eye.

Risk: PRK is the lowest risk followed by Epi-LASIK. Flap procedures have a mildly higher risk with Intra-LASIK felt to be safer than LASIK.

Outcomes: depending on the study there have been some differences found between procedures in small studies, but overall the long term results appear to be similar between all types of laser vision correction techniques.

Laser: each center will have a particular type of laser which may have the capacity to do customized treatments. The laser application will be essentially the same at a center regardless of the procedure type.

When given a choice between a low risk flap based procedure with a return to work within a few days and a lower risk no-flap procedure, some people will choose the more rapid return to work. Others will choose the lower risk treatment and accept the longer recovery. What it comes down to is each individual's choice.

Flap Procedures: LASIK versus Intra-LASIK

The difference between these two procedures is the method of flap creation. With LASIK the flap is created using a standard microkeratome. With Intra-LASIK the flap is created using an ultrafast femtosecond laser. With both techniques the laser reshaping step is done the same way using an excimer laser.

The rate of complications with standard LASIK is very low but can include a variety of intra-operative and post-operative complications as mentioned earlier. A more in depth discussion can be found in Chapter 10. Generally the standard microkeratomes create a flap depth of 120 microns to 180 microns. More recently there are SBK (sub-Bowman's keratomelieusis) microkeratomes that can create thin flaps that are 90 to 120 microns, as thin as those created by the femtosecond laser.

Intra-LASIK is felt to be safer than standard LASIK due to the fact that the flap can be visualized while it is being created, the femtosecond laser is less likely to result in an irregular flap, a more planar flap is created (meaning the inner and outer surfaces are parallel), and a more perpendicular side cut is created with Intra-LASIK. These factors are felt to improve the safety of the flap creation step compared to standard microkeratomes and also are felt to reduce the risk of flap shift with post-operative trauma. Since the femtosecond laser is very new compared to standard microkeratomes there are no large scale studies to date that compare the complications with the two systems.

LASIK and Intra-LASIK both rely on a suction ring to secure the cornea and to create a planar flap. A planar flap is important in reducing the optical impact of the flap on the overall correction. Most surgeons will use an algorithm, an adjustment, when they do the calculations to create the correction that is to be entered into the laser that will include an adjustment for the flap if necessary. Algorithms will vary between surgeons, lasers, and techniques.

The suction ring raises the intraocular pressure and causes the vision to dim or black out. For LASIK the vision may be affected for about thirty seconds and there will be a sensation of pressure along with a vibration from the microkeratome. With Intra-LASIK the vision will dim out for up to a minute, there is a heavy pressure during that time, and the femtosecond laser is quiet.

With either method once the flap is made the remainder of the procedure is essentially the same. The flap is lifted and the excimer laser is used to reshape the cornea. The excimer laser has a loud snapping sound and creates a smell like burnt hair. When the laser reshaping, also called laser ablation, is complete the flap is replaced using a sterile irrigating solution to rinse off debris and smooth the flap.

For both LASIK and Intra-LASIK the recovery is similar. Most people will return to their usual activities within a day or two. There may be some stinging or burning in the first twenty-four hours and increased dry eye for up to several weeks in some cases. For most people the vision may continue to sharpen and the night vision will improve over weeks to months.

No-Flap Procedures: PRK and Epi-LASIK

PRK is the original laser vision correction surgery which was first performed by Dr. Margueritte MacDonald in 1988 in the US and in 1990 by Dr. John Van Westenbrugge at the Gimbel Eye Centre in Canada. With the advancement of excimer laser technology in recent years the risk of haze or scarring has been dramatically reduced, and PRK has become more popular again due to the excellent long term results and safety profile.

All of the no-flap procedures, also known as surface ablation, involve removing the outer cells of the cornea called the epithelium. Basic eye anatomy can be found in Chapter 7. For PRK the epithelium is usually removed with either an automated brush or using a dilute alcohol solution to soften the epithelium for easy removal. With Epi-LASIK an epikeratome is used to remove the epithelium. The epikeratome is similar to the microkeratome but uses an epithelial separator with a suction ring to stabilize the eye during the epithelium removal step. Originally when Epi-LASIK was developed, the epithelial sheet was replaced following the laser reshaping. As this technique has developed most surgeons feel that recovery is faster if the epithelium is removed.

The main difference between PRK and Epi-LASIK is the method of epithelium removal. Once the epithelium is removed the laser reshaping is done in the same way with the excimer laser.

Advocates of Epi-LASIK feel that the epikeratome produces a cleaner edge at the perimeter of the treatment zone than can be achieved with the brush. Epi-LASIK is also done without the use of alcohol which might slow healing to some degree. Among surgeons who favor no-flap procedures there is some debate as to whether or not Epi-LASIK provides more rapid healing as compared to PRK. Since Epi-LASIK is a newer technique there are no large scale studies to compare these two techniques.

Epi-LASIK requires the use of a suction ring so there will be pressure on the eye and the vision will dim or black out for about thirty seconds. This is similar to the sensations with LASIK and Intra-LASIK. With PRK there is no suction ring so that step is not required. The excimer laser reshaping is the same as described above for flap procedures.

With both PRK and Epi-LASIK a bandage contact lens is placed at the end of the procedure to help with comfort and will remain in place for three to five days. Most people will need approximately one week off work or driving. The majority of people find that the first three days are the worst

Chapter 5: How to Choose Between PRK, Epi-LASIK, LASIK, or Intra-LASIK

for discomfort and blurred vision. Pain following no-flap procedures generally varies from mild to moderate, three to six on a scale up to ten. A variety of medications both oral and eye drops are given to guard against infection and to help with comfort. By about a week most people are back to their usual activities although the overall acuity and night vision will improve over a few weeks to a few months.

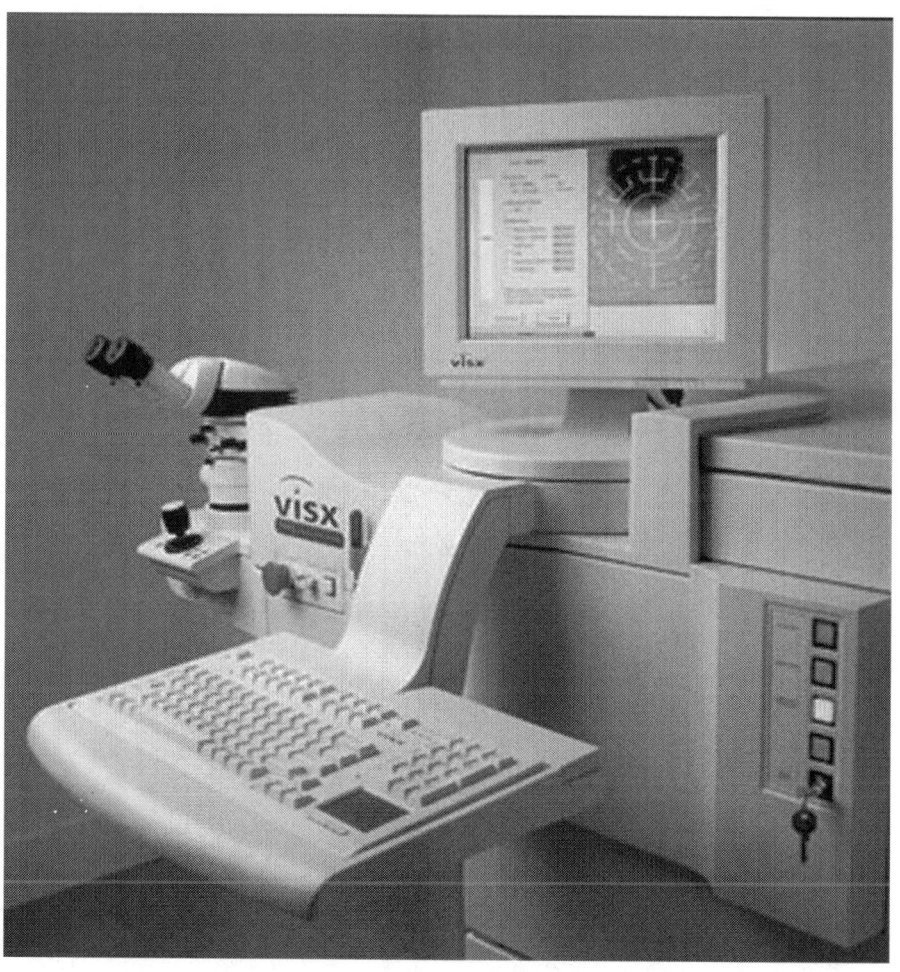

Some excimer lasers have the capacity to use iris recognition to do a rotational adjustment for the precise placement of custom wavefront treatments.

Custom, Wavefront, and Standard Laser Treatments

Regardless of whether or not a flap is made, the laser application can be standard, custom, or wavefront treatment. A standard laser treatment will correct the astigmatism and nearsightedness or farsightedness. A wavefront treatment requires that an aberrometry map be measured before surgery. Aberrometry measures the individual variations of an eye called higher order aberrations. The difference between the wavefront treatment and standard treatment is similar to the difference between an off the rack suit and a tailored suit. The wavefront laser treatment will correct the individual aberrations in addition to the astigmatism and nearsightedness or farsightedness.

There are some lasers that will also do a more refined variation of a standard treatment which preserves the shape of the cornea. The cornea is naturally flatter on the outer edges; this shape is called aspheric. An aspheric laser treatment will preserve the cornea's natural flattening in the periphery which is thought to assist in reducing side effects like glare and halo.

Types of Laser Treatments

Standard: standard usually refers to a simple treatment of your prescription including the hyperopia, myopia, and astigmatism.

Custom wavefront: custom will usually refer to individualized laser treatments that use wavefront technology to measure the aberrations in the eye for use in a refined individualized correction.

Aspheric: refers to a blended zone in the peripheral cornea which will maintain the natural shape of the cornea which is flatter in the periphery.

Chapter 5: How to Choose Between PRK, Epi-LASIK, LASIK, or Intra-LASIK

In general if you qualify for a true wavefront treatment, it is likely to give better results with respect to quality of vision. There are some reasons why you may not qualify for a wavefront treatment. Your surgeon should discuss with you what your options are and which treatment is best for your individual case.

Other Acronyms: ASA, KASA, Intralase, LASEK and more

In the effort to attract more clients various acronyms have been used over the years to describe the techniques of LASIK, Epi-LASIK, Intra-LASIK, and PRK. Most of these other acronyms are a variant of one of these four basic techniques. It is likely readers will encounter acronyms that are not on this list as new variants are constantly being created.

Other Acronyms Used For Laser Vision Correction

ASA/AST: Advanced Surface Ablation/Advanced Surface Treatment refers to PRK or Epi-LASIK combined with a wavefront laser treatment.

KASA: Keratome Assisted Advanced Surface Ablation refers to Epi-LASIK in which an epi-keratome is used in combination with a wavefront or custom laser treatment.

LASEK: Laser In Situ Epithelial Keratomeleusis is another word for Epi-LASIK but usually referring to alcohol assisted epithelial removal.

Intralase: this is a brand name for one of the femtosecond lasers used to create the flap for Intra-LASIK.

SBK: sub-bowman's keratomeleusis is a thin-flap LASIK technique.

At this time, regardless of the acronym used the majority of treatments are a variation of one of the flap or no-flap techniques combined with a standard or custom excimer laser correction.

How to Choose

It is important to educate yourself about the procedures available. Find a surgeon and laser center you trust, and have an assessment to see if you are a good candidate for laser vision correction. There may be reasons why a particular procedure may be recommended for you. Be sure to ask a lot of questions so that you understand the risks and benefits of the procedure that is recommended. Since surgeons have differing opinions about which procedure offers the best outcome, it can be helpful to get more than one opinion.

Choices you may have to make will include:

- flap versus no-flap procedure
- custom versus standard procedure
- distance target or mono-vision (if you are forty or older)
- which surgeon and center

When you have an assessment you will usually be given printed information and often you will watch an informational video. It may be helpful to look at the websites of the centers that you are considering. Additional information can be found on websites such as those listed in Chapter 1.

Keep in mind that if you are following blogs or discussion groups for refractive surgery that the stories you may read may not necessarily apply to your case. Your regular optometrist or ophthalmologist may also be a good source of information. If you have been seeing an eye care provider for a number of years they will know your individual eye conditions and will likely be aware of the laser vision correction surgeons in your area.

Summary

If you are a candidate for laser vision correction you will need to learn more about risks and benefits of the procedures available to you. Although uncommon, there is a possibility of complication and you will need to be comfortable with the choices you make. Your choice of procedure should be made with the assistance of a qualified surgeon's advice following your laser vision correction assessment.

CHAPTER 6: WHAT TO EXPECT FROM LASER VISION CORRECTION

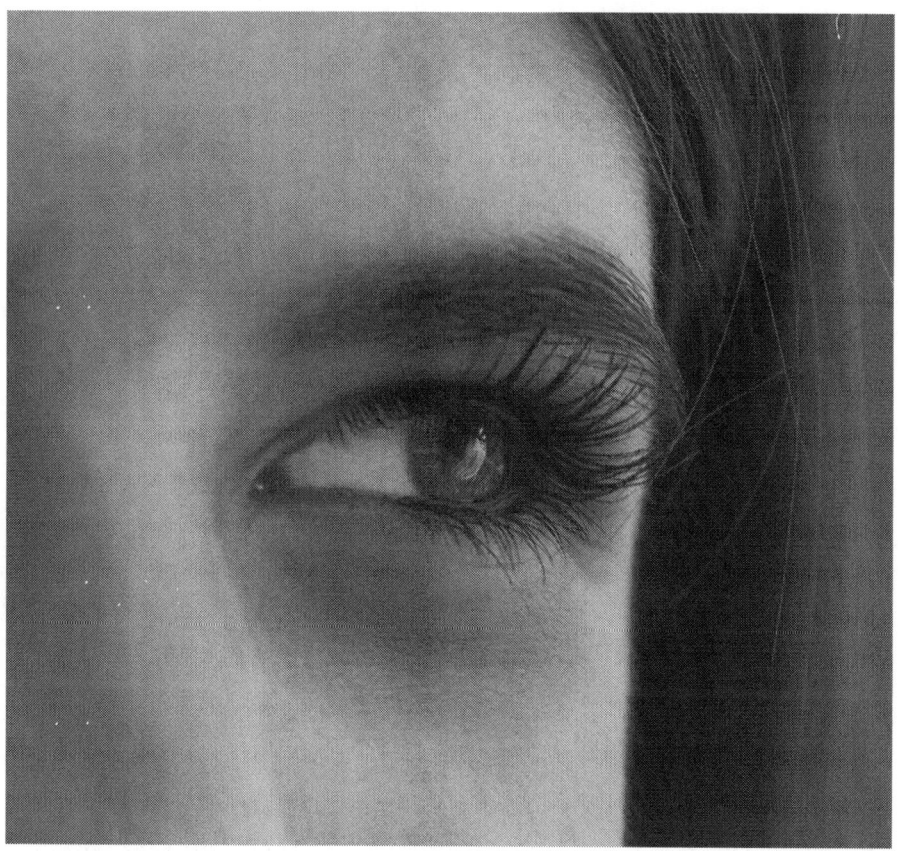

Over 28 million people have undergone laser vision correction. Of those who have had laser vision correction, over ninety-five percent of people are satisfied with their outcome. This figure has been reported to have remained stable over the past decade. According to the American Society of Cataract and Refractive Surgeons (ASCRS) less than 1 in 10,000 US LASIK patients are unhappy with their results.

While less than 1 in 10,000 is a small number, with millions of surgeries being done worldwide each year the number of unsatisfied patients has reached a high enough number that the FDA in cooperation with the ASCRS has launched a quality of life study in 2008. This study aims to identify factors which will enhance patient care. One factor that seems to correlate with higher satisfaction is having the right expectations before surgery.

Why isn't there a guarantee?

Laser vision correction is a surgical procedure. No matter how skilled the surgeon or how careful the assessment prior to surgery, there are a variety of factors that can lead to less than satisfactory results. The surgeon and the laser center can offer to continue follow up and testing or perform additional corrective procedures if possible, but they can not change healing processes or predict all possible outcomes. In some cases additional surgery can not be done or may make the situation worse. Most surgeons and laser center staff are committed to providing the best possible outcomes and highest level of safety, but even with the highest level of skill and knowledge it is not possible to guarantee results.

What kind of things might happen?

Specific information about complications of laser vision correction can be found in Chapters 8 to 11. Most complications can be divided into intra-operative (something that happens during surgery), early post-operatively (something that happens within a few hours to a few days after the procedure), and later post-operatively (something that might happen months or years after treatment).

Five to fifteen percent of people might need a second treatment or enhancement to achieve their best vision. This is not considered a complication but is due to differences in healing and response to the laser. In most cases it is advisable to wait up to six months to make sure the measurements are stable. If there is only a small amount of residual correction measured or if it is noticed only when covering the other eye, enhancement may not be recommended. The higher the original measurements the more likely a second

Chapter 6: What to Expect from Laser Vision Correction

treatment might be needed. Farsighted (hyperopic) treatments are more likely to need an enhancement.

For all of the laser vision correction surgeries the excimer laser is used to reshape the corneal tissue. In rare cases there can be things that might affect the treatment and cause irregularities on the cornea which might result in poor vision. This is called irregular astigmatism and can also be caused by healing factors after surgery.

Causes of irregularity intra-operatively can include things such as water spots on the mirrors inside the laser system or debris or irregularities on the cornea surface that are not taken care of prior to firing the laser. Some lasers have a protective shield in place when the laser isn't firing which protects the mirrors from splashes. Calibration will often require firing the laser onto a clear plastic plate to be inspected for beam irregularities. Many laser centers also have a policy of visual inspection of the mirrors between cases. Routine maintenance also would include inspections and cleaning of critical parts such as mirrors. The surgeon is looking at the surface of the cornea at all times and will clear off the corneal surface to make sure there is a smooth surface on which to apply the laser treatment.

Irregular astigmatism is uncommon following laser vision correction and in most cases if it is the result of an intra-operative complication it can be treated with additional surgery. If it is a result of irregular healing, called ectasia, it may not be treatable with more surgery.

For both flap and no-flap treatments it is possible to have a corneal scratch or abrasion either on top of the flap or outside the treatment area of no-flap treatments. These abrasions might delay the healing but in most cases will not affect the long term results.

For flap procedures like LASIK and Intra-LASIK, intra-operative complications can occur while the flap is being made. These complications can include partial flaps, buttonholes, or irregular flaps. A flap complication is very uncommon with LASIK and is reported to be even more uncommon with the Intra-LASIK. If a minor flap complication happens during surgery, in some cases the excimer laser re-shaping can still be done. For more serious flap complications the flap must be left in place or repositioned without doing the laser treatment. In many cases it will be possible to have future procedures to fix the problem. In rare cases there may be a permanent irregularity that can affect the vision and might not be treatable or may require a corneal transplant.

Early post-operative problems are very uncommon but can include infection or inflammation (redness, swelling, or early scarring) with both flap and no-flap treatments. For all types of laser vision correction an examination will be recommended one to three days after treatment in order to check for these types of early problems. Antibiotic and anti-inflammatory drops are also prescribed to prevent these early complications. In the majority of cases, with early detection at the first post-treatment visit, these problems can be treated with a change in medication. In very rare cases an additional surgery might be needed, or in extremely rare cases there may be a permanent loss of vision. To reduce the risk of infection you will be most likely advised to avoid swimming or hot-tubs and to take other precautions for the first few days to a week following surgery.

For flap treatments there is a risk of flap shift which is most likely to happen within the two days after treatment. For that reason many centers will advise wearing protective shields while sleeping and avoid eye rubbing for a few days following LASIK or Intra-LASIK. The flap will usually not be shifted by a bump to the head or by vigorous exercise, but may shift if there is direct contact with the cornea. In rare cases a flap shift can happen even months or years following surgery if there is a direct blow to the eye. In most cases the flap can be repositioned in the laser suite. Safety glasses are always recommended for those activities such as using power tools where safety glasses are normally worn. Safety glasses should be worn whether you have a flap treatment, no-flap treatment, or no surgery.

Chapter 6: What to Expect from Laser Vision Correction

Late post-operative complications are very uncommon. In addition to late flap shifts due to trauma, in very rare cases the cornea may become unstable due to a condition called ectasia. There has been an enormous amount of debate and research into what causes ectasia. From the information available at this time it appears that risk factors include thinning the cornea too much, corneal irregularities such as keratoconus before surgery, and family history of corneal diseases like keratoconus.

Ectasia is more common after flap procedures such as LASIK but has been reported following no-flap treatments such as PRK. Further laser surgery can not be done if ectasia develops. Treatment of ectasia consists of glasses or specialized contact lenses and in severe cases corneal transplant may be needed. Fortunately this condition is extremely rare and will most likely become even less likely to occur as more research is being done on the corneal response to laser vision correction.

The overwhelming majority of people are satisfied with their results of laser vision correction. Even though the risk of a bad outcome is very low, it is important to read all of the information provided to you by your surgeon including the surgery consent form. Understanding the risks will help you make the best choice about whether to have laser vision correction and about which treatment is best for you.

What to do if a complication occurs

The first thing to do is to talk to your surgeon. It can be helpful to understand what happened and what to expect as far as recovery or future need for additional surgery. Be sure to ask as many questions as you need to in order to understand what the treatment plan will be.

Possible Outcomes Following a Complication

It may resolve on its own: some complications such as swelling, inflammation, or over correction will resolve over time with healing.

Treatment with eye drops may be effective: for mild infections or inflammation treatment with drops may resolve the situation.

Additional surgery may correct the problem: for situations such as a shifted corneal flap or an irregularity of the corneal surface, additional surgery may correct the problem.

Specialized contact lenses: for serious complications that can not be treated with additional surface surgery or drops there are specialized contact lenses that can be used to optimize visual acuity.

Corneal transplant or other specialized treatments: for serious complications such as corneal irregularity from ectasia a corneal transplant or newer techniques such as corneal crosslinking may be recommended to aid in vision recovery.

If you undergo laser vision correction and are one of the few who have a complication of surgery, you must be patient with your recovery. In many cases the eye must be stable before any further treatment can be done. It may be up to six months or longer before further treatment can be done. Sometimes interim eyeglasses or

Chapter 6: What to Expect from Laser Vision Correction

contact lenses might be needed. In some cases a second opinion from a qualified surgeon is helpful to confirm your treatment plan is appropriate and to investigate other options if available.

In the very rare cases where there is a complication that can not be treated, optimize your vision with glasses or contact lenses. There are ophthalmologists and optometrists that specialize in customized corrections for people with more complex needs.

Will I be able to see 20/20?

The majority of people will be able to see 20/20 after laser vision correction. A few people will be better than 20/20. A few may not be 20/20. Vision of 20/20 is considered normal and describes the line on the eye chart that most people can see from 20 feet. Better than 20/20 would be 20/15 or less commonly 20/10. Worse than 20/20 would be 20/25, 20/30, 20/40 and so on. The laser vision correction is intended to reshape the cornea to create a zero optical power for distance. For many people this will result in 20/20 vision. This concept will be discussed in more detail in Chapter 7. The result of corneal reshaping is to allow you to see as well without glasses or contact lenses as you did before surgery.

If you were not correctable to 20/20 before surgery, laser vision correction will not improve your best corrected vision. For example if you have amblyopia which is sometimes called a lazy eye and your best vision has been 20/40 then you would not expect to see better than 20/40 even with a perfect laser vision correction result. Some eyes do not have the capability to see 20/20. If you need bifocal glasses or wear reading glasses when you wear contact lenses, you will need reading glasses for close work following surgery unless you choose the monovision option in which one eye is left nearsighted to aid in reading.

It can take a number of days or weeks and sometimes months for the healing to be complete. Over that time frame the overall sharpness of vision can improve, night vision will improve, and in some cases an enhancement can be done once the vision stabilizes. Be sure to talk to your surgeon about what to expect following your laser vision correction.

What to expect before the day of surgery

The details of the pre-operative assessment are explained in more detail in Chapter 3. You can expect the assessment to last about two to three hours during which time a number of specialized tests and measurements will be performed. Dilation drops will be used in order to allow for more accurate measurements of your prescription as well as to allow for inspection of the peripheral retina. Following dilation drops you may not be able to drive for up to several hours so you should arrange for alternate transportation. Your surgeon may request additional testing if necessary.

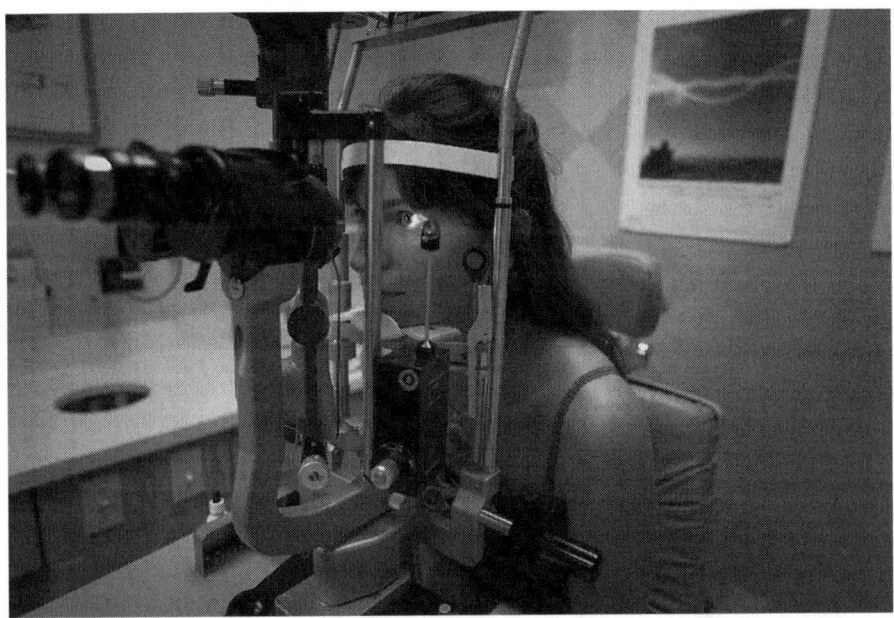

A slit lamp is a specialized microscope that allows your ophthalmologist to do a detailed examination of the surface and the interior structures of the eye.

Chapter 6: What to Expect from Laser Vision Correction

In most centers you will be shown an information video or DVD and given written materials as well. You will most likely meet with your surgeon or in some centers you will meet with an optometrist who will examine you and discuss the details of your eye health with you. In most cases you will discuss with your surgeon or the optometrist which procedures you may qualify for and if there are any specific recommendations for treatment. This is your chance to ask any questions you may have about laser vision correction in general and about your case in particular. It can be helpful to bring a list of questions and to write additional questions down as you go through the assessment.

If you decide to book a surgery then additional information including a surgical consent form will be provided to you. Be sure to read the consent thoroughly and ask any additional questions if needed before signing. The surgical consent is a legal document. Signing the consent means that you have read and understood the contents of the consent.

You will most likely be provided with instructions and some prescriptions for eye drops prior to the day of surgery. Be sure to follow all instructions carefully. For example in most centers the instructions will include not to wear perfume or cologne. This is very important due to the fact that these scents can affect laser performance. In some cases people who have not followed instructions have been required to wash in the bathroom and change into a scrub top before surgery will be done.

What to expect on surgery day

It is essential to arrange for a driver on the day of surgery and for one or more follow up visits. If you come without alternate transportation on the day of surgery your surgeon will likely have to cancel your surgery due to the fact that a sedative is usually recommended and your vision will be blurry immediately after surgery so you can not drive yourself home from the surgery. Most centers will require you to be accompanied by another adult when you leave the center after surgery. Following the pre-operative instructions will optimize your safety and vision results.

You will generally be expected to pay your surgery fee when you check in, before any surgery is done. In some cases repeat testing may be performed. After this you will probably meet with surgery center staff to confirm your procedure type and which eye (or both). Staff will go over additional information with you about what to expect during and after surgery as well as instructions for post-operative eye drops.

In most cases you will have had a chance to read the surgery consent before the day of surgery. If not then you will need to take the time to read the consent thoroughly before you sign it. If you have met your surgeon previously and have no additional questions, then an oral sedative will be offered. In general the sedative is a good idea as it will help you relax during surgery, however it is not mandatory to take a sedative.

If you have not previously met with your surgeon then you will have a chance to speak to the surgeon for a few minutes before signing the consent and taking the sedative. Often the surgeon will examine your eyes one more time with a specialized instrument called a slit lamp. If you do have any last minute questions it can be helpful to write them down to bring with you on the day of surgery.

Once you are brought into the laser suite you may be asked to wear a hair cover and sometimes shoe covers. The laser suite is a clean environment and extraneous dust or hair may pose a risk of infection. Anesthetic (freezing) drops are used to numb the surface of the eyes. The lids will not be frozen so you will have sensation on the lids throughout the procedure. For some procedures a sterile plastic drape will be put around the eye (sticks onto the skin with adhesive). For all of the procedures a small wire speculum is used to hold the eyelids open. The speculum will give you a tugging or pulling sensation on the lids, especially if you blink or squeeze the lids.

Chapter 6: What to Expect from Laser Vision Correction

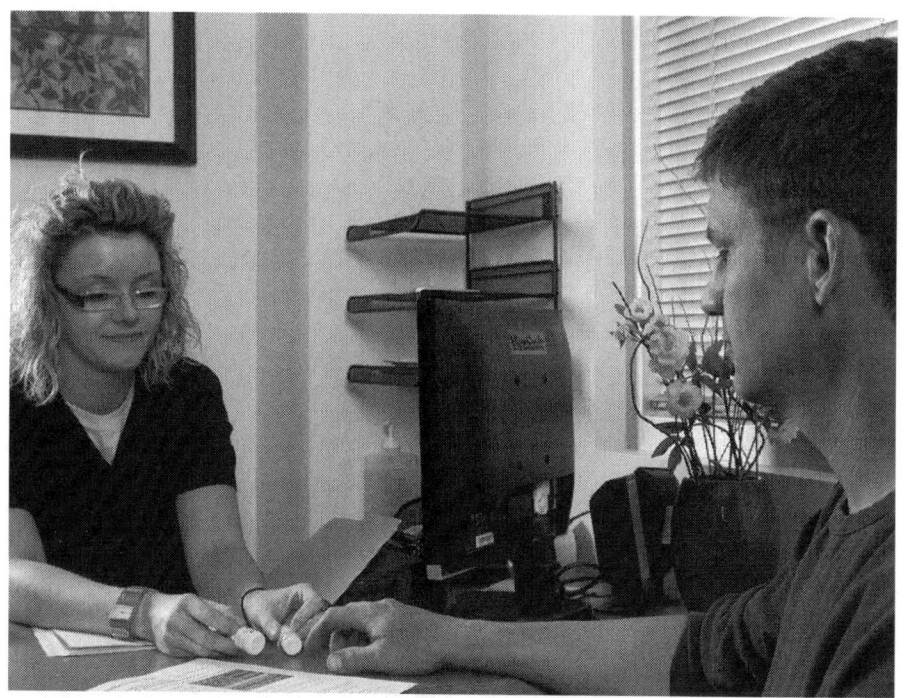

You will usually meet with a counselor at your assessment and again on the day of surgery to discuss the details of your care. Photo by Dave Best.

The details of each procedure will be explained in Part II of this book. All of the procedures are generally between five and fifteen minutes per eye from start to finish. One eye is done at a time and for all of the procedures you can expect that the vision will be blurry immediately following the treatment. The blurred vision will be similar to looking through fog, dirty glasses, or glasses smeared with Vaseline.

For flap procedures you can expect the vision to be clearing over about twenty-four hours such that you may be legal to drive. Most people will experience some stinging, burning, light sensitivity, or gritty feeling for the first twenty-four hours.

For no flap procedures the vision and comfort will worsen somewhat over the first two days before it starts to improve.

What to expect in the first week

Depending on which surgery you have you will need to return for follow up appointments one to three times within the first few days, and possibly at one week after the treatment.

For no-flap treatments a bandage contact lens will remain in place for the first three to four days. There will be a moderate to significant amount of discomfort ranging from a feeling of sand in the eyes to stinging and burning requiring pain medication. Light sensitivity is common after all laser vision surgeries. Some people may need to rest in a dark room for the first few days. Usually the contact lens will be removed in three to four days and you may be legal to drive within four to seven days. Legal to drive is not 20/20 so driving and other activities may need to be modified for several days to a few weeks. It is important to be patient with your recovery in the first weeks following a no-flap treatment.

For flap treatments many patients are legal to drive within the first twenty-four hours. Some patients may experience light sensitivity or mildly blurred vision for a few days to a few weeks.

For any laser vision correction treatment the two eyes may respond differently. One eye may have a more rapid recovery of vision or may have more discomfort during the healing phase. Sharpness of vision, dry eye, and night vision will continue to improve for several weeks to several months. Be sure to discuss any concerns with your eye care provider at your follow up visits.

What to expect in the first few months

After the first week for both flap and no-flap treatments there will usually be a few follow up visits within the first six months. Follow up for specific treatments will be discussed in more detail in Part II of this book.

Chapter 6: What to Expect from Laser Vision Correction

In general these follow up visits do not require dilation and will be relatively quick. Once you are in the legal range for driving you will likely be able to drive yourself to most of these follow up appointments. In rare cases there may be a need to be dilated, and your provider should advise you if you need a driver.

For no-flap treatments it may take a few weeks to a few months for your vision to gradually sharpen up. For both flap and no-flap treatments symptoms such as dry eye, night vision problems, and fluctuating vision will continue to improve over several weeks to several months. Patience is critical as this gradual improvement occurs.

If you have a complicated case then your need for follow up may be increased and there may be more testing required. In a small number of cases if there is a significant over or under correction there can be a need for an interim pair of glasses or contacts if there is a need to wait for the prescription to stabilize before considering retreatment or enhancement surgery. In most cases it is advisable to wait up to six months to make sure the cornea has stabilized prior to performing additional laser treatment. Over this time side effects like dry eye or glare and halo at night are likely to improve.

The goal of laser vision correction is to be functioning as well after the healing period following surgery as you did before surgery with corrective lenses. It is important to work with both eyes together and avoid comparing eyes as there can be natural differences in healing between them. An enhancement or retreatment may be recommended if the correction is stable and if you are bothered by residual correction when working with both eyes together.

For many people, once the follow up care is completed they may have routine eye examinations every two years or so depending on their age and other medical conditions. A few people will find that they have some persistent dry eye or mild worsening of night vision compared to before surgery, although the majority of people will find their eye comfort and vision will be similar to what it was like before surgery with glasses or contact lenses.

Summary

It is helpful to know what to expect during and after surgery. Proper expectations can reduce the stress and anxiety of undergoing surgery and will increase your chance of satisfaction with the outcome of laser vision correction.

PART II: **LASER VISION CORRECTION IN DETAIL**

CHAPTER 7: EYE ANATOMY

In order to understand laser vision correction surgery it helps to understand the basic anatomy of the eye and how vision works. Often the analogy of a camera is used in order to describe the various functions of specific parts of the eye.

Eye Structures

Lids and lashes:	normal lid function is important in eye health.
Extraocular muscles:	there are six muscles surrounding the eye that allow the eyes to move and to work together.
Tear film:	the layer of tears that covers the cornea plays an important role in clarity of vision.
Conjunctiva:	the thin mucous membrane which covers the outside of the sclera as well on the inner surface of the upper and lower lid; inflammation or irritation of the conjunctiva leads to a red eye.
Sclera:	the thick white tissue that surrounds the eye.
Cornea:	the most anterior (forward) structure, the cornea is like the clear windshield of the eye.
Anterior chamber:	underneath the cornea is a chamber filled with a liquid called aqueous.
Iris:	the iris is the colored part of the eye which functions like a shutter in a camera to let in more or less light.

Pupil:	the pupil is the space within the central iris border; the pupil generally looks black due to the fact that light does not usually exit the pupil except on rare occasions such as a camera flash when the light reflects back (red reflex).
Lens:	the lens of the eye is located behind the iris and focuses light on the retina.
Vitreous:	the cavity behind the lens is filled with a gelatin like substance called the vitreous.
Retina:	the retina lines the back of the eye and functions like film in a camera to capture images. The central part of the retina is called the macula and is responsible for color vision and sharp central vision.
Optic nerve:	the optic nerve carries the information from the retina to the brain.
Brain:	there are several structures within the brain that are essential for proper visual functioning.

Although laser vision correction is performed on the cornea, it is important that all of the structures are healthy and functioning properly in order to have good visual acuity.

The process of vision involves light rays that first travel through the clear corneal structure. The cornea bends the light to variable degrees depending on the corneal curvature. The light then passes through the aqueous which is the water-like substance in the front of the eye. The light rays will then encounter the lens of the eye. The lens of the eye is like the lens of a camera and in younger people the lens can change shape to change the focal point of the light. This process is called accommodation. This focus ability

Chapter 7: Eye Anatomy

becomes weaker with age until sometime after the age of forty a reading glass or bifocal lens will be needed for close work. After the light passes through the lens it then travels through the vitreous gel that fills the space between the lens and the retina. When an object is in focus the light rays are focused on the retina. The focal points in nearsightedness, farsightedness, and astigmatism are discussed in Chapter 2.

The retina is like film in a camera and receives the incoming light. The light is translated via complex chemical reactions into nerve impulses which travel from the retina through the optic nerve and to the visual areas of the brain. The messages received in the brain are organized into what is perceived as vision. Normal vision is considered to be 20/20. Vision of 20/20 means that a person can read a specific line on a standard eye chart at the standard distance of twenty feet. Vision that is worse than 20/20 will have a number larger than 20 as the second number. For example the bigger lines on the eye chart are usually 20/25, 20/30, 20/40, 20/50 and so on. Some people may read better than 20/20 such as 20/15 or rarely 20/10. Some eyes do not have the capacity to see 20/20 due to a variety of factors. Some investigators believe that 20/5 is the best vision that is possible even with perfect optics in the rest of the eye due to the limiting factors of the retina. Most standard eye charts will stop at 20/15 or 20/10 since it would be extremely rare to have the ability to read better than those lines. The metric standard for 20/20 is 6/6 which refers to vision measured at 6 meters. When assessing vision it is important to have standardized distances and equipment.

There are other factors that influence vision such as contrast sensitivity (the ability to distinguish between shades of gray), color vision, stereo vision, and peripheral vision. It is possible to be able to read 20/20 but still not be seeing properly if these other functions are not working properly. Visual acuity on the standard eye chart is the usual method used to assess vision. Depending on symptoms and the eye exam findings, additional vision tests can be done to investigate problems with the other areas of visual functioning. For the majority of

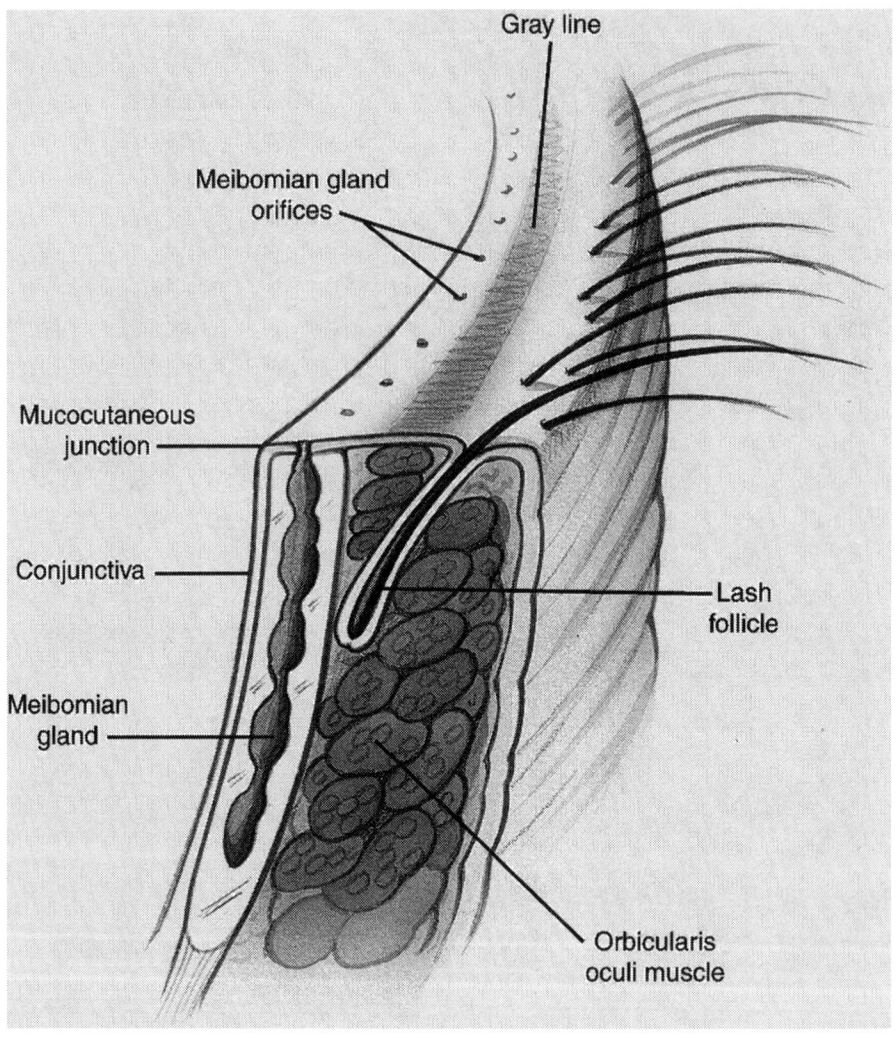

The lids are important in protecting the eye and in maintaining a healthy tear film. © 2009 American Academy of Ophthalmology

people these additional tests may not be needed, and a simple standard acuity is sufficient to assess visual functioning.

Lids and Lashes

The lids provide an important protective structure for eye health. If the lids do not close properly due to injury or disease, laser vision correction may not be recommended. Problems with the lashes such as in-turned lashes should also be addressed before considering laser vision correction. There are a variety of conditions which can affect lid function ranging from congenital (things you are born with) conditions to injury or disease.

Common Lid Conditions

Blepharitis:	dysfunction of the oil glands in the lids that can lead to dry irritated eyes and inflammation of lid margins.
Ectropion:	turning out of the eye lid, most commonly the lower lid, can lead to tearing and irritation.
Entropion:	turning in of the lids which can cause the lashes to touch the surface of the eye leading to chronic irritation.
Lagophthalmos:	lids that don't close completely. This can happen for a number of reasons and often leads to dryness and irritation.
Ptosis:	drooping of the upper lid; many be congenital or acquired.
Trichiasis:	lash mis-direction; often causes chronic irritation.

The most common lid condition that can affect the outcome of laser vision correction is blepharitis. Blepharitis is related to skin conditions such as rosacea or seborrheic dermatitis. Blepharitis causes plugging of the oil glands in the eye lids and can lead to inflammation of the lid margins. It is a common cause of dry eye and lid discomfort. Treatment of blepharitis may include warm compresses for three to five minutes twice per day, artificial tears, and lid scrubs with dilute baby shampoo once per day. In more severe cases antibiotic ointments or oral antibiotics can be helpful.

The lids also contain the drainage structures responsible for draining excess tears. In some people a blockage of the drainage ducts will lead to tearing. In severe dry eye these ducts can be intentionally closed with punctal plugs or cautery. Your surgeon should discuss with you any lid conditions that may affect your comfort or vision following surgery.

Extraocular Muscles

Imbalance of the eye muscles can lead to double vision. In some cases a prism in eyeglasses may be needed. If you need a prism eye glass then laser vision correction may not be advisable. If you have had a previous eye muscle imbalance but can wear contact lenses comfortably and without double vision then laser vision correction may be safe for you.

It is possible to trigger a worsening of an underlying eye muscle imbalance with laser vision correction. If you have any current problem with double vision or a previous history of eye muscle imbalance you should discuss it with your surgeon before surgery.

Tear Film

Although not a true anatomic structure, the tear film is critical in maintaining eye comfort and clarity of vision. The tear film is composed of oil, mucous, and a water-like fluid. If the tear film composition is disrupted by conditions such as blepharitis then the eye will be prone to dryness and irritation. There are also medical conditions that can lead to a decrease in tear production. Any tear film dysfunction should be treated before undergoing laser vision correction. Dry eye is one of the most common side effects of any laser vision correction surgery, so if you have dry eye before undergoing surgery it is likely to be worse following surgery if not treated appropriately.

Treatment of Dry Eye

Artificial tears: there are a variety of artificial tears available over the counter that vary in thickness up to gels and ointments. In general tears that contain preservatives can be used up to eight times per day, and preservative free tears can be used as often as every few minutes.

Punctal plugs: temporary or permanent closure of tear drainage ducts.

Warm compresses: soaking the eye lids with the eyes closed with a warm wet cloth twice per day can thin out oil secretions and help tear composition.

Flax & fish oil: oral supplementation with a combination of flax oil and fish oil can aid in tear production; they act in two different ways to help dry eye.

Medicated eye drops: in severe cases of dry eye the use of topical steroid or cyclosporine drops may be necessary. Laser vision correction should not be considered if you suffer from severe dry eye.

Humidifiers: humidifiers in the home or work space can help dry eye.

Frequent breaks: taking a break about every 15 minutes from computer or reading for about 15 to 20 seconds to look at a distant object and blink several times can help your own tears wet the eye more effectively. The blink rate is significantly reduced when concentrating on close work.

Be sure to discuss any dry eye concerns with your surgeon before undergoing laser vision correction. A poor tear film can compromise the results of both flap and no-flap treatments. With proper treatment mild to moderately dry eye can be improved. If you suffer from dry eye you may have to use drops or other treatments every day. Just as with dry skin, a daily regime is sometimes necessary to maintain a healthy tear film.

Conjunctiva

The thin outer membrane that covers the sclera and the inner part of the upper and lower lid forms an important protective structure for the eye. Anything that irritates the eye from dryness to allergies to infection will make the eye red. If the eye is inflamed and red it is a good idea to identify the cause and treat before considering laser vision correction.

For chronic conditions such as allergies or dry eye it is important to have the eye quieted down before surgery. For flap procedures it is especially important not to rub the eyes as this may shift the flap following LASIK or Intra-LASIK. Regardless of whether or not you have laser vision correction, eye rubbing will increase the chances of the inflammation to become chronic and can lead to thinning of the cornea. If you have a habit of rubbing your eyes you should work with your eye care provider to break this habit and control your symptoms with appropriate treatments before you consider any excimer laser treatment.

Causes of Red Eye

Infection:	conjunctivitis (pink eye) is usually viral in adults and can follow a common cold. Surgery should be postponed until the infection is cleared.
Dry eye:	treatment of dry eye is discussed earlier in this chapter.

Allergies:	it is advisable to have allergy symptoms controlled before undergoing laser vision correction.
Eye rubbing:	even small amounts of rubbing causes worsening inflammation and redness. With significant eye rubbing, swelling of the lids and thinning of the cornea may result. Rubbing is a risk for flap shift after LASIK or Intra-LASIK.
Medicated drops:	over-use of some drops such as the "get the red out" formulas can lead to chronic redness. Other prescription medications may also lead to a red eye. Some people are sensitive to preservatives in eye drops.
Lid or lash conditions:	there are a number of lid conditions that can lead to a red eye; some examples are listed earlier in this chapter.
Pterygium:	a triangular benign corneal growth resulting from wind and sun exposure.
Inflammation:	conditions such as episcleritis or iritis can lead to a red eye.

Eye injuries or eye surgeries that cause scarring may affect which treatments might be recommended. Larger scars on the conjunctiva might interfere with the suction rings that are used in LASIK, Epi-LASIK, and Intra-LASIK. If you have a condition involving the conjunctiva, your surgeon should discuss your options and how your condition might affect the outcome of laser vision correction.

Conditions Involving the Sclera

Fortunately there are not too many conditions that affect this important structure. The sclera is a tough layer of connective tissue that surrounds the eye. Serious trauma, some eye surgeries, and inflammation can involve this layer of the eye. Inflammation of this layer is called scleritis and can be a complication of rheumatoid arthritis. People with a history of scleritis would not be candidates for laser vision correction.

If you have had significant eye trauma or eye surgery you should discuss this with your surgeon. Irregularities of the sclera might interfere with the suction ring that is used for Epi-LASIK, Intra-LASIK, and LASIK.

Corneal Anatomy

The cornea is composed of several clear layers starting the most anterior (furthest toward the outside) epithelial layer. The corneal epithelium is made of epithelial cells which rest on a clear membrane called Bowman's membrane. The epithelium has the capacity to regenerate quickly which is why no-flap techniques are effective. The epithelial layer that is removed with the no-flap treatments of PRK and Epi-LASIK heals within three to four days. The epithelium also has the capacity to fill in irregularities on the corneal surface. As healing is occurring over weeks to months following no-flap treatments the epithelial healing has a smoothing effect which improves sharpness of vision.

If the Bowman's layer underlying the epithelium is injured the epithelial cells may not stick as well which can lead to recurrent corneal erosions (abrasions). Injuries to Bowman's layer can occur with a sharp injury to the cornea such as being scratched with a fingernail. Recurrent corneal erosion also can be an uncommon side effect of laser vision correction surgery. People with this condition may awaken in the morning with a spontaneous painful corneal abrasion. There are some disorders such as map-dot-fingerprint or hereditary corneal dystrophies which can affect this layer of the cornea. Disorders or previous injuries that affect Bowman's membrane might disqualify you from flap based treatments of LASIK and Intra-LASIK and from Epi-LASIK.

The majority of the cornea is made of clear tissue called stroma. The corneal stroma can be involved in deep corneal

Chapter 7: Eye Anatomy

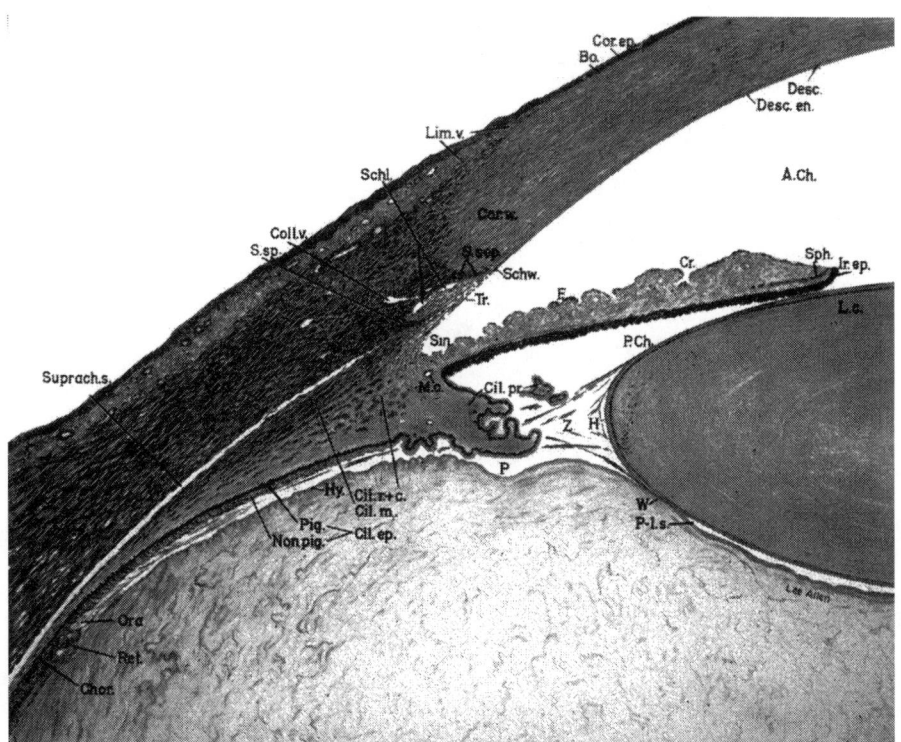

The corneal epithelium is the outermost layer of cells that is removed to prepare the surface for excimer laser treatment during PRK and Epi-LASIK. The corneal epithelium is indicated by "cor ep" in this microscopic cross-section of the eye. © 2009 American Academy of Ophthalmology

injuries or hereditary corneal dystrophies. PRK and Epi-LASIK remove only the thin epithelial portion of the anterior corneal stroma, leaving the underlying stroma untouched. The flap which is created in LASIK and Intra-LASIK will weaken the anterior stroma to a greater depth since once the flap is cut into the corneal stroma. Once the flap is cut it no longer contributes to the structural integrity of the cornea to the same degree. For this reason flap procedures pose more of a risk for corneal instability or ectasia.

The innermost layer of the cornea is called the endothelium which is composed of a layer of cells which adhere to thin layer of connective tissue called Descemet's membrane. The endothelial cells are critical in pumping excess fluid out of the cornea. Injuries or disorders which damage the endothelium or Descemet's membrane can lead to corneal swelling which causes poor vision. There is some debate as to whether laser vision correction should be offered to people with conditions that affect this layer of the cornea as it may be a risk for corneal swelling following surgery.

Corneal Layers

Epithelium: the outermost layer of cells which regenerates quickly. The epithelium is removed for no-flap treatments and regrows in three to four days.

Bowman's membrane: the epithelial cells are attached to this thin membrane. Damage to Bowman's can cause recurrent abrasion or scars.

Corneal stroma: the stroma makes up the largest part of the cornea. Flaps created with LASIK or Intra-LASIK cut into this layer of the cornea.

Endothelium: the innermost cells of the cornea responsible for pumping excess fluid out of the cornea. Endothelial damage can lead to corneal swelling.

Descemet's membrane: the endothelial cells attach to Descemet's membrane. Damage to Descemet's membrane can lead to corneal swelling.

A normal cornea is usually between 500 microns and 600 microns. Corneal thickness will affect which treatments will be appropriate for you. A thin cornea may be a contraindication to a flap procedure such as LASIK or Intra-LASIK. Your surgeon should discuss with you any concerns related to corneal thickness and which treatments may be best for you. If your cornea is very thin, laser vision correction may not be recommended due to the risk of corneal instability or ectasia due to over thinning.

Chapter 7: Eye Anatomy

The normal cornea will have a regular shape. Abnormal corneas or corneas that may be prone to irregularity may have an irregular shape. Corneal conditions such as keratoconus or pellucid degeneration are considered contraindications for laser vision correction. There are more subtle changes that may indicate a "forme fruste" or a precursor to keratoconus or pellucid. Corneal mapping should be performed as part of the pre-operative assessment.

Dry eye and contact lens wear can interfere with corneal mapping. For this reason you will be advised to leave your contacts out for two days to two weeks for soft lenses and up to four weeks for rigid gas permeable lenses. If your eye is dry or you have worn your contact lenses recently you may need to have the maps repeated after treatment of dryness or a longer time out of your lenses.

For custom wavefront treatments it is of particular importance to have good maps as this information will be used to create the customized laser treatment. If obvious irregularities exist you may not qualify for surgery. For more subtle irregularities you may still qualify for a no-flap treatment, and your surgeon should discuss these map findings with you.

Anterior Chamber

The anterior chamber is the space between the inside of the cornea and the iris. The anterior chamber is filled with a watery substance called aqueous. There are only a few conditions that will cause problems in the anterior chamber. The most common problems encountered will be iritis and a shallow anterior chamber.

Iritis is an inflammation of the inside of the eye which causes cells to accumulate in the anterior chamber and in more severe cases in the vitreous. Iritis is also sometimes called uveitis. When the anterior chamber is viewed with magnification at the slit lamp in a patient with iritis, it looks like a shaken snow globe. If you have a history of iritis then laser vision correction is not recommended as you may be at a higher risk of vision threatening complications.

A shallow anterior chamber is sometimes noticed at the assessment examination. A shallow chamber means that the space between the iris and the cornea is smaller than average. This can also be called a narrow angle. This condition results in a higher risk of a sudden increase in intraocular pressure due to angle closure glaucoma. A normal pressure may range up to about 22 mm Hg, and can go as high as 70 mm Hg in an acute angle closure attack. Angle closure is an emergency requiring emergency laser iridotomy and treatment with topical and oral medications. If you are identified as having a narrow anterior chamber, your surgeon may recommend you undergo a prophylactic laser iridotomy before undergoing laser vision correction.

Injury or surgery that involves the anterior chamber may pose a risk for laser vision correction. Your surgeon should discuss any abnormalities of the anterior chamber with you before surgery.

Iris

The iris is the colored part of the eye and is located inside the eye between the lens and the anterior chamber. The iris is analogous to the shutter in a camera and is responsible for pupil size changes. There are some conditions that can cause scarring or irregularities of the iris. In most cases iris irregularities are due to significant inflammation such as can occur in iritis, or can result from trauma. Depending on the cause of the irregularity you may still qualify for laser vision correction.

The unique individual patterns of the iris are like a fingerprint. This feature is utilized in iris recognition used in wavefront treatments. The iris is recognized and a cyclotorsion (rotation) adjustment is made if necessary to precisely match the wavefront treatment pattern to the cornea.

Pupil Size

The pupil is the space in the center of the iris. The pupil looks dark due to the fact that light enters but does not usually exit the eye. Infrequently there may be light reflected back out of the eye from the retina such as occurs with "red eye" with a camera flash.

Over the past decade there has been a lot of debate over the role of pupil size and night vision complaints following laser vision correction. There has not been a definitive study to demonstrate that large pupils are truly a risk factor for night vision problems following surgery. If you have pupils that are larger than eight mm in dim light it is possible that you may be at a higher risk for night vision problems like glare and halo in dim or dark light. Although rare, this can be a particular problem for night driving and is difficult to treat. Treatment includes night driving glasses or mild constricting drops for night driving. These treatments may improve but not eliminate night vision symptoms. In addition, large pupils may not qualify for wavefront custom treatments.

Very small pupils may pose a problem if you are interested in wavefront custom treatment. For some systems a pupil size of less than five millimeters may disqualify you from a wavefront treatment. The parameters may differ between systems so you should discuss your individual case with your surgeon prior to surgery.

Regardless of pupil size, most people find that the night vision takes longer to improve. Be prepared to limit your night driving for a few weeks to a few months following surgery. For the majority of people who have laser vision correction the night vision will return to the way it was before surgery. If you have poor night vision or glare and halos at night prior to treatment you can expect it will be worse for a period of time before returning to baseline. For higher corrections and flap procedures the night vision can take up to a year to return to baseline. While there are a few people who find their night vision to be improved following surgery, you should not be expecting an improvement in night vision as a result of laser vision correction.

For some wavefront treatments the pupil size must be between five and seven millimeters in size. These requirements are due to the fact that if the pupil is too large then the iris recognition step is difficult. If the pupil size is too small then there may not be enough wavefront data to do the treatment.

Conditions of the Lens

The lens of the eye is responsible for the ability to focus from far to near. As a natural result of the aging process, the ability to focus becomes weaker with age. This is called presbyopia. The majority of people will need reading glasses over their contact lenses, bifocal or multifocal contact lenses, or bifocal or progressive spectacles sometime between the ages of forty and forty-six.

If you are considering laser vision correction and are in this age range or older, you may want to consider the option of monovision. In monovision corrections one eye is corrected for distance and the other eye for near vision. Monovision can be simulated with contact lenses or a trial frame (a set of lenses that can be put into a special frame to hold the lenses). A trial frame is not quite as good a test as contact lenses but may allow demonstration of monovision in the office it you don't wear contact lenses. If you are forty or older you should ask your surgeon about monovision. If both eyes are corrected for distance in this age range you will need reading glasses immediately or within a few years following laser vision correction.

If you choose monovision, the goal will be to give you the widest range of functional vision without having to put your reading glasses on. There are some people with monovision that do not wear glasses. Others may need glasses for night driving or other demanding distance activities. For very fine close work there are some people who will use reading or near vision glasses. A monovision trial with contact lenses will give you the best trial of this option.

Another condition that may affect the lens is cataract. Cataract is a clouding of the lens of the eye. A few people are born with lens changes which is called congenital cataract. Congenital cataracts are usually very stable and if they do not interfere with vision they may not interfere with laser vision correction.

Chapter 7: Eye Anatomy

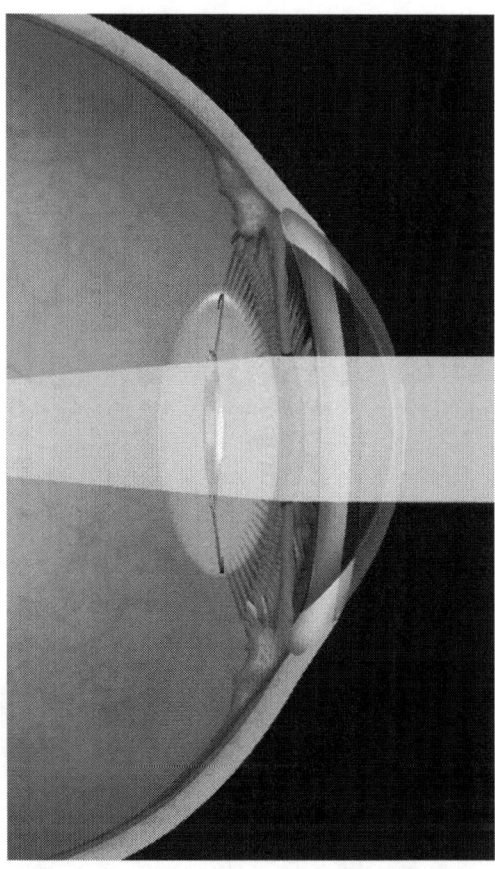

The lens inside the eye is responsible for focusing the light as it enters the eye. Lens implants for cataract surgery are placed in the same location as the native lens.

Age related cataracts may affect the prescription and can cause the vision to be reduced even with the best corrective lenses. If you have cataracts then laser vision correction may not be recommended. If you have a stable prescription and your cataracts are not advancing you may still qualify for laser vision correction. If you have cataracts it is possible you may need cataract surgery in the future, and your laser vision center should provide you with pre-operative measurements that may be necessary for future cataract surgery. In some cases such as someone over the age of fifty-five a cataract surgery may be a better option. If you have cataracts your surgeon will discuss this with you before recommending laser vision correction.

Vitreous

The space behind the lens is filled with a jelly like substance called the vitreous. When you are young the vitreous is like a solid block of gelatin. As part of the aging process the vitreous can become liquefied and form clumps or strings which appear in the vision as floaters. Inflammation of the eye can also lead to vitreous floaters which will appear like a string or dots moving across the vision.

There are very few vitreous conditions that would prevent laser vision correction, however vitreous floaters will not be improved with corrective surgery. Although unlikely, it is possible that procedures such as LASIK, Intra-LASIK, and Epi-LASIK which all use a suction ring could cause additional floaters. Any sudden change in the number or size of floaters should be reported to your eye care provider within a day or two.

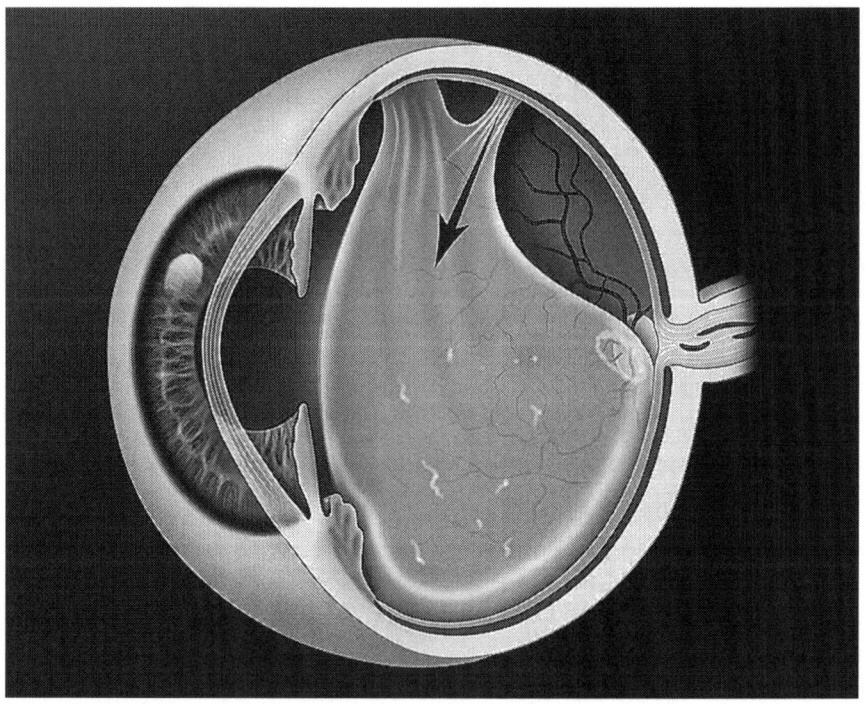

The back of the eye is filled with a gel called "vitreous". Some people develop floaters which are condensations of the vitreous gel which occur with age. © 2009 American Academy of Ophthalmology

Retinal Conditions

The retina lines the back of the eye behind the vitreous cavity. The retina is analogous to film in a camera. The retina captures the images which are transported through the nerve fiber layer of the retina to the optic nerve and to the visual areas of the brain. The center of the retina is called the macula and is responsible for color vision as well as sharp central acuity. The peripheral retina provides peripheral vision and is important for vision in low light. Nearsighted people are more at risk for peripheral retinal breaks, detachments, or weak areas of the peripheral retina.

If the retina is damaged, laser vision correction will not correct any resulting vision problems. Any existing retinal conditions need to be stabilized before considering any laser vision correction. A complete examination of the retina should be performed as part of the preoperative assessment including a dilated retinal exam. In some cases a co-managing optometrist or ophthalmologist may perform this dilated examination.

If there are any concerns about the retina, additional testing or referral to a retina specialist may be required before undergoing laser vision correction. There have been rare reports of retinal tears, retinal detachment, or retinal hemorrhages following laser vision correction.

Optic Nerve

The most common condition to affect the optic nerve is glaucoma. There are several types of glaucoma with the common result of thinning of the optic nerve rim and loss of peripheral vision. In many cases the pressure inside the eye may be elevated, but it is possible to have glaucoma with a normal pressure. This is called normal pressure or low pressure glaucoma. The result of advanced glaucoma is tunnel vision or blindness. There is some debate about the safety of using a suction ring such as is used in Epi-LASIK, Intra-LASIK, or LASIK in people with glaucoma due to the stress of raised intraocular pressure on an already compromised optic nerve.

If you are taking drops for glaucoma it may affect healing. Other less common conditions that can involve the optic nerve include optic neuritis and conditions affecting blood flow to the eye such as ischemic optic neuropathy. If you have been diagnosed with glaucoma or other optic nerve disease you would need to discuss this with your surgeon.

The Brain

Proper functioning of the visual areas of the brain is critical in visual performance. There are numerous disorders that can affect the brain causing visual disturbances. One of the more common disorders that is seen in people who are interested in laser vision correction is called amblyopia, also known as a "lazy eye". An eye that is "lazy" does not develop the proper connections with the brain and will have poor vision compared to a normal eye. Unfortunately laser vision correction can not improve an amblyopic eye beyond what the best acuity is with glasses or contacts.

Other conditions of the brain that can affect vision include stroke, and tumors. If you have a stable condition with some vision impairment you should discuss your condition with your surgeon before considering laser vision correction.

The brain is also important in the ability of adjust to changes in vision. For example some people will easily adjust to monovision where one eye is corrected for distance and the other for near vision. Other people can not tolerate this imbalance.

For people that are very particular about their glasses or contact lenses laser vision correction may not be advised. It is not possible to guarantee that the two eyes will be exactly equal in acuity or that it will be exactly the same as the previous glasses or contacts. If you have trouble adjusting to new prescriptions you may not be a good candidate for laser vision correction.

Another factor affecting satisfaction following laser vision correction is the ability to cope with adversity. Although uncommon, complications may happen which delay the recovery of vision or in rare cases might cause a permanent loss of vision. If you suffer from untreated depression or anxiety it may be more difficult for you to cope with a poor outcome. Don't forget, the risk of laser vision correction is very low but it is not zero.

Eye Disease

There are far too many disorders and diseases that can affect the eye to be completely covered in a short paragraph, but below are some of the more common conditions.

Common Eye Diseases and Disorders

Cataract: clouding of the lens of the eye more common in older patients. Refractive lensectomy may be a better choice if you have cataracts.

Glaucoma: as discussed earlier under the optic nerve section glaucoma is not always a contraindication to eye surgery.

Corneal dystrophy: corneal dystrophy such as keratoconus or pellucid degeneration are considered contraindications for vision correction surgery.

Dry eye: significant dry eye should be discussed with your surgeon.

Blepharitis: inflammation and plugging of the oil glands of the lids that leads to increased risk of dry eye and irritation.

Iritis: inflammatory disorders such as iritis can pose a risk for laser vision correction.

Herpes simplex:	herpes simplex can reactivate with laser surgery.
Keratoconus:	corneal dystrophies such as keratoconus and pellucid degeneration are contraindications to laser vision correction.
Macular degeneration:	deterioration of the central retina that leads to a decrease in central vision. This can not be corrected by laser vision correction.
Lazy Eye/squint/ strabismus:	different names for a crossed eye or an out-turned eye ("wall-eye) which may affect candidacy for laser vision correction.
Presbyopia:	age related need for reading glasses.

These are just a few conditions that may be found at an assessment. The goal of a pre-operative examination is to identify any disorders that might present a threat to vision or an increased risk of laser vision correction.

Summary

It is helpful to have an understanding of eye anatomy in order to accurately understand the risks and benefits of laser vision correction. Your usual eye care provider and your surgeon are resources for information and education about your individual eye health.

CHAPTER 8: PRK

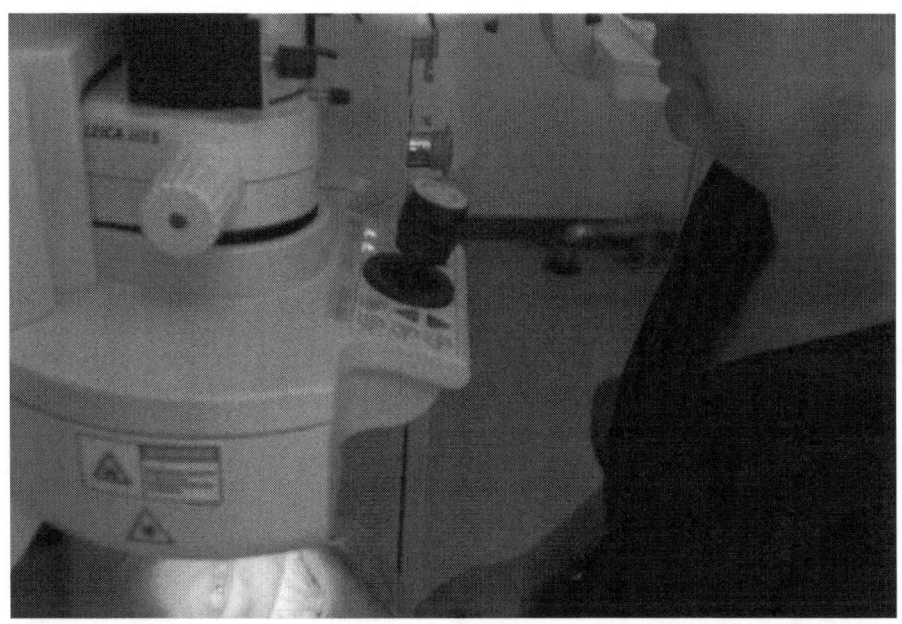

Photo by Dave Best.

Photorefractive keratectomy (PRK) is the oldest laser vision correction technique that is still in use. PRK has withstood the test of time since first introduced by Dr. Margueritte MacDonald in 1988. Over twenty years later it is still offered by many refractive surgeons. Phototherapeutic Keratectomy (PTK) is a variant of PRK in which the excimer laser is used to treat irregularities of the cornea. PTK is sometimes used to treat irregularities following PRK.

How is PRK done?

For PRK the eye is frozen with anesthetic eye drops. The surface of the eye is frozen but the lids are not. It is normal to feel sensation on the lids. A lid holder (speculum) is placed on the eye to hold the lids open. The other eye may be covered with a patch. If you blink or squeeze, you will feel the lid holder tug or pinch on the eyelids. In most cases a sedative will be offered. Although the sedative will not make you sleepy, it is a good idea to take the sedative as it will help the procedure go more smoothly.

The surface epithelial cells are removed from the surface of the cornea with a brush or with dilute alcohol. If a brush is used you may feel some pressure and a vibration. With the dilute alcohol you will likely feel a little pressure followed by rinsing with saline. With either technique the vision will become more blurry. You will usually be instructed to keep looking straight ahead (towards the ceiling since you will be supine) or to look at the target light which will usually be red/orange. It is helpful to avoid squeezing the other eye. If you can think about opening both eyes between blinks it will help to look straight with the eye that is being treated.

If you feel faint, sweaty, or unwell it is important to tell your surgeon. Although uncommon, it is possible to faint in the middle of a procedure. This usually will not cause any problems but can delay the surgery. If you let your surgeon know you don't feel well, it is easy to take a few minutes to put a cold cloth on your forehead, take a break, or drink some juice or water. In some cases a simple repositioning is helpful, such as putting a pillow under the knees to help your back or other measures. The more comfortable you are the more quickly the procedure will be completed.

Once the surface of the cornea is prepared the laser will be aligned. You will be instructed to look at the target light. It is normal that the target light will look blurry and it will look like it is moving from your heart beat and breathing. It can be helpful to look through the light as if you are looking at the ceiling to avoid trying to follow the light around. If you look away the laser will stop, and the surgeon will realign the laser before resuming. Usually there is no effect on the outcome if this happens. If the laser has to be repeatedly aligned, there may be an increased chance you will need an enhancement. Many lasers have an eye tracker which will follow small movements of the eye that are called saccades.

Chapter 8: PRK

When the laser fires there will be a loud snapping noise like a bug zapper. There is usually a smell like burnt hair or branding. This smell is the result of the particles released as the corneal tissue is ablated (evaporated) by the excimer laser. Some lasers have a suction device to help vacuum up these particles, but it does not usually eliminate the smell completely. After the laser treatment some drops are placed along with a bandage contact lens to protect the cornea as it is healing.

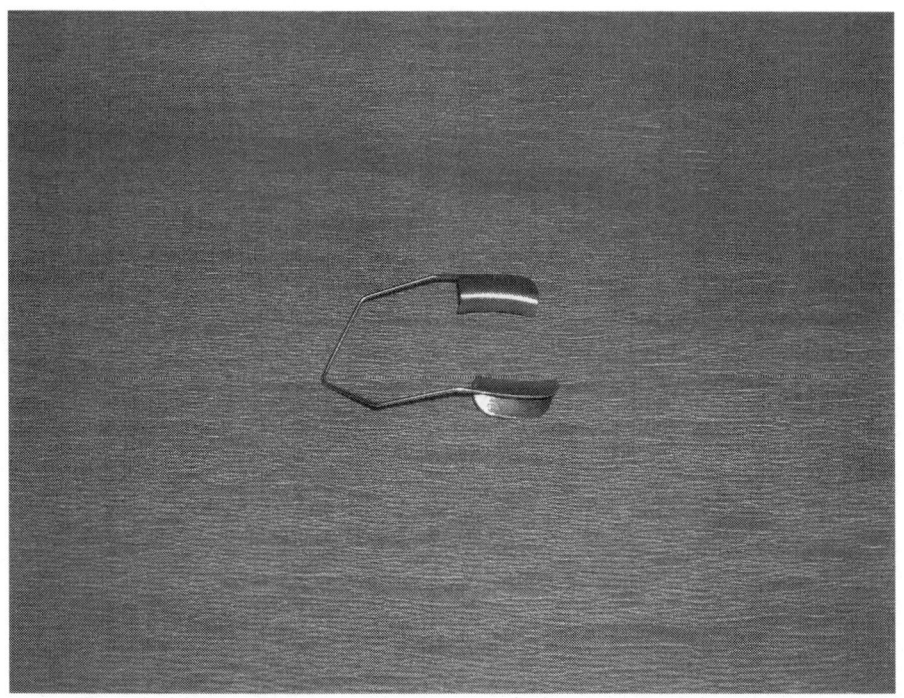

A small lid holder called a lid speculum will be used to prevent the eye from closing during PRK.

Healing

In general the bandage contact lens will stay in place for three or four days. In rare cases it may take longer for the surface epithelial cells to heal. For most people the discomfort and vision will get worse over the first two days.

There are many people who have mild discomfort, like sand under the contact lens. There are some people who become very light sensitive and have significant discomfort. If you have significant discomfort following PRK it may be necessary to stay in a dark room and take the pain medications that are provided.

You should plan to take it very easy for three to four days following PRK. It is helpful to spend as much time with the eyes closed as possible for the first few days following PRK. There will be antibiotic and anti-inflammatory drops that will be prescribed following surgery. It may be beneficial to use preservative free artificial tears for the first few days after PRK. Preservatives can slow healing or cause irritation.

Often a freezing drop is also provided. The freezing drop can slow healing so should be used sparingly. If it is the middle of the night and you are trying to sleep you should use the freezing drop. It will give you about twenty minutes of relief which may be enough to get back to sleep. If the contact lens falls out you should replace it with a new lens. If you are not comfortable putting a contact lens in your eye then you should call your surgeon.

Many centers will check your eyes the day after surgery. This is a safety check to make sure there are no signs of infection or inflammation. If everything is healing as expected, which means the comfort and vision will worsen over the next two days, there will be a check on the third or fourth day after surgery. In most cases the contact lenses will be removed on the third day, but there is no guarantee. Everyone heals differently so there are a few people who may have the contact on longer.

Once the contact lens is removed you may be legal to drive. Legal to drive is usually a few lines away from 20/20. The driving standards will vary between states and provinces. It is possible that you may not be legal to drive for up to seven to ten days following PRK. You should not resume driving until your surgeon tells you that you meet the legal

Chapter 8: PRK

vision requirements. In some cases you may meet the legal requirements but may not feel comfortable driving. When scheduling your surgery it is helpful to have at least a week off work following PRK.

Many people find that they have some vision fluctuation for four to eight weeks. You may have to take more frequent breaks from computer or reading, and you may have to limit your night driving during this time. Frequent artificial tears may help. For most people the overall sharpness of vision, dry eye symptoms, and night vision will improve over this time. It is important to be patient with your recovery and plan to take breaks or limit night driving if needed.

Over the next four to six months you may be advised to continue taking medicated drops to avoid regression (healing back towards your original prescription). Post-operative dryness, night vision problems, and overall sharpness of vision will continue to improve over several weeks to months after surgery. If you have any concerns you during your healing you should discuss it with your surgeon.

Post-operative Care

In an uncomplicated PRK case you will usually have a post operative check on the first day following surgery and then within a few days after surgery to remove the bandage contact lens. Once the bandage contact lens has been removed and you are in the legal range for driving, there will usually be a post-operative check once a month for three to six months depending on the healing response.

Complications

PRK is very safe and has been performed in North America for over twenty years. However, the risk in not zero. During surgery it is possible that there could be loose epithelium outside of the treatment zone that could result in delayed healing. It is also possible that there could be a decentration of the laser treatment or other factors that could lead to irregularity of the surface of the eye. In most cases this type of irregularity can be corrected with additional surgery.

Post-operative complications of PRK are also uncommon.

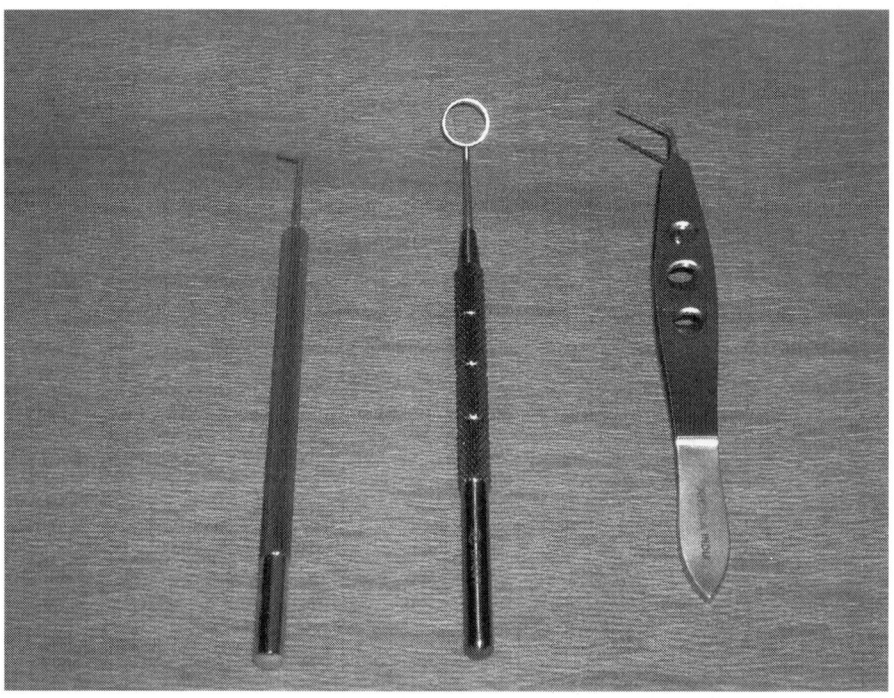

For alcohol assisted PRK a small circular well is used to keep the solution in a precise area for removal with a blunt spatula. Forceps are used for insertion of the contact lens following laser treatment.

Post Operative PRK Complications

Infection: it is possible that infection might develop within the first few days following surgery. In most cases infection can be treated.

Scar/haze: with newer lasers it is very uncommon to have significant scar or corneal haze.

Under or overcorrection: a small percentage of people will over or under respond to laser vision correction. Once the correction has stabilized in most cases an enhancement can be done.

Recurrent erosion: in some cases the corneal epithelium develops a weakness following surgery that can result in a spontaneous abrasion. In many cases this can be treated with topical drops.

Regression: in some cases the eye heals back in the direction of the original prescription. This can be corrected by a retreatment.

Ectasia: in very rare cases corneal instability can result from laser vision correction surgery.

Dry eye: dry eye is the most common side effect of any laser vision correction.

Night vision changes: although uncommon, glare and halo at night may worsen following any type of laser vision correction surgery.

The list above contains the most common possible complications. Other uncommon complications are decentered treatment and irregular astigmatism. It is not possible to predict all possible complications, but pre-operative testing is intended to identify people who may be at high risk for complications of laser vision correction.

In most cases complications of laser vision correction will either resolve over time or may be treated with medications or further surgery. Many people do feel they are more sensitive to airborne irritants due to the fact the eyes are no longer protected by corrective lenses. In some cases corrective lenses may be needed to improve vision. In rare cases there may be complications following PRK that may lead to a loss of vision that may not be treatable.

Enhancement (retreatment) after PRK

PRK involves the treatment of the corneal surface. The cornea is living tissue and so can heal and respond differently in different individuals. For this reason a percentage of people will need a second treatment, known as an enhancement, for their best vision. In all cases the correction needs to stabilize before additional surgery can be done. This may take six months or longer in some cases. A few people may have a need for a corrective lens for driving while they are waiting for enhancement. For many people the amount of residual correction is low enough or affects only one eye so they may be able to drive and do usual activities without corrective lenses while waiting for the cornea to stabilize.

Reasons for Retreatment after PRK

Regression:	healing back towards the original correction.
Under-response:	a residual amount of correction can remain if the corneal tissue does not respond as expected to the laser treatment.

Over-correction: the intended correction can result in an over-correction if the cornea responds more than anticipated to the laser treatment.

Irregular astigmatism/ scarring/haze: with newer lasers it is uncommon to have significant haze, scarring, or corneal irregularities after PRK.

Some people have a strong healing response which can lead to regression which causes the eye to heal back towards the original prescription. Regression is more common in higher corrections and in far-sighted corrections. Most surgeons will recommend a mild steroid drop be used for three to six months following PRK to reduce the chance of regression. The steroid drop is usually recommended on a tapering schedule such as four drops per day for the first month then three drops per day for the second month and so on. The schedule might be modified in order to slow healing further or in some cases reduced more quickly to encourage more rapid healing. While on a steroid eye drop the eye pressure should be checked periodically since some people will develop high eye pressure due to steroid drops. If regression occurs you will have to wait up to six months or longer for the correction to stabilize before considering an enhancement.

There are some cases where the amount of tissue removed with the excimer laser might be less than intended. This is known as an under-correction or an under-response. There are several theoretic reasons for this including corneal hydration and ambient humidity. Laser centers will have their excimer laser in a climate controlled room with a constant temperature and humidity to avoid fluctuations in laser energy that is delivered to the cornea. Surgeons will usually use a standard surgical technique in order to avoid variations in corneal hydration during PRK.

The correction data is often altered based on factors such as degree of correction and age in order to compensate for the likelihood of under-response in certain cases. For higher corrections a special topical medication called mitomycin-C may be used at the time of surgery to slow healing and prevent regression. In spite of all these measures there are some people who will under-respond to the treatment. In these cases there will be residual correction measured immediately after surgery. It is still necessary to wait for up to six months before enhancement surgery to make sure the correction is stable.

Similar to under-correction, the same factors described above can lead to an over-correction which is sometimes called an over-response. When over-correction happens the measured prescription will be opposite the original correction. For example you may have been near-sighted (myopic) before surgery and then far-sighted (hyperopic) immediately following surgery. Alternatively if you were far-sighted to start with, you may be near-sighted immediately following PRK. In these cases your surgeon may modify your post-operative drops to encourage faster healing. In some cases regression or healing back towards the original correction will lead to self correction of a small over-correction over the weeks and months following surgery. For PRK a mild over-correction is expected in the first month or so since the cornea usually settles a little back towards the original prescription. For a significant over-correction it may be necessary to wear reading glasses or distance glasses while waiting for the prescription to stabilize.

The rate of enhancements varies from about five to fifteen percent depending on how high the starting prescription. The higher the prescription the more likely you might need a second treatment for your best vision. It is very uncommon to do more than one enhancement, although in rare cases it may be necessary. Repeated enhancements are usually not recommended. If the prescription is unstable there may be other factors such as cataracts or diabetes that are having an effect on the eye. There may be some cases when your surgeon may recommend against any further surgery and you may be back into glasses or contact lenses. Although this is uncommon you and your surgeon need to weigh the risks and benefits of each repeat surgery before deciding to proceed.

More complicated treatments may be needed if haze, scarring, or irregular astigmatism results from PRK surgery. In these cases a smoothing treatment can sometimes be done with the laser called phototherapeutic keratectomy or PTK. If you need PTK your surgeon should discuss the treatment plan and expectations with you before retreatment.

Summary

PRK is an excellent option for most people who qualify for laser vision correction. This technique has been in use for over two decades and has very good long term results and stability. It is a lower risk compared to flap procedures due to the simplicity of this technique. The risk is never zero. For some people with thinner corneas, surface treatments such as PRK may be the only option for laser vision correction. You should discuss your options with your surgeon and be sure to have all your questions answered before deciding if PRK is a good option for you.

CHAPTER 9: EPI-LASIK

Epi-LASIK is a newer variant of surface PRK. The original idea was that the epithelial flap would be created with dilute alcohol (also called LASEK) or with the Epi-keratome and then the epithelial flap could be repositioned after the laser treatment to enhance healing. In practice, keeping the epithelial flap increases healing time. In more recent years surgeons have found that removing the epithelial flap improves healing. PRK and Epi-LASIK are both no-flap surface treatments. The main difference between PRK and Epi-LASIK is in the epithelial removal step.

How is Epi-LASIK done?

Drops are used to freeze the surface of the eye. The drops do not freeze the lids so there will be sensation on the lids during the treatment. As with all corneal eye surgeries a lid holder (speculum) is placed on the eye to hold the lids open. The other eye may be covered with a patch. If you blink or squeeze you will feel the lid holder pinch or tug with each blink. It is a good idea to take a sedative as it will help the procedure go more smoothly by allowing you to hold steady during the treatment.

For Epi-LASIK the epikeratome is used to remove the epithelium. The epikeratome uses a suction ring to stabilize the eye. While the suction ring is in place on the eye the vision will dim or black out for about 30 seconds. During this time you will feel pressure and a buzzing sensation. The epikeratome uses a separator which oscillates at a high rate to push the epithelium off.

The vision will become more blurry as the procedure progresses. For the majority of the treatment you will either be asked to look straight ahead, which will be towards the ceiling since you will be supine, or to look at the target light which will usually be red/orange. It is helpful to avoid squeezing the other eye. Thinking about opening both eyes

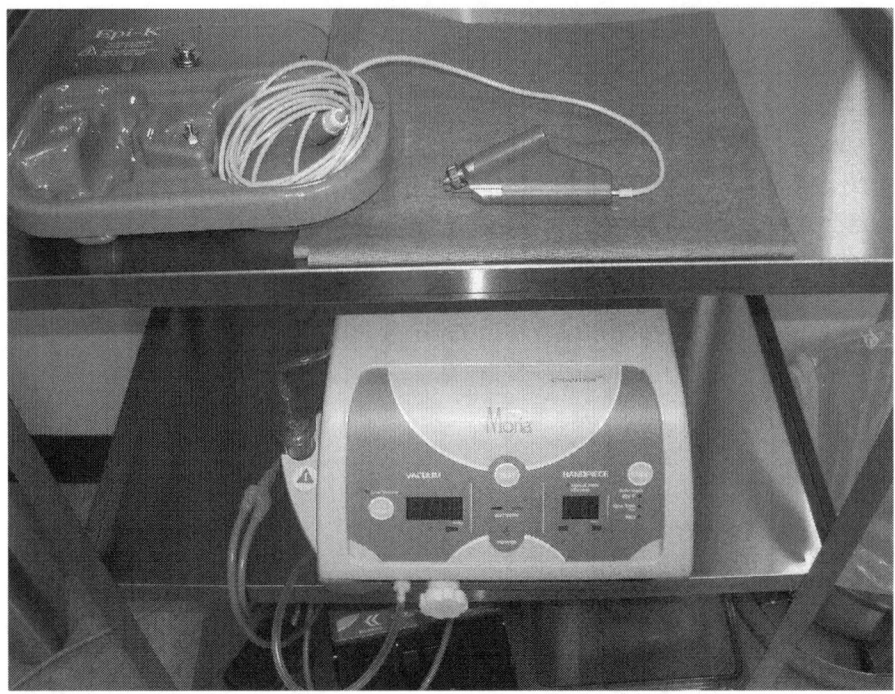

The epikeratome has a power-source which drives a small motor in the handpiece which in turn drives an oscillating separator to remove the corneal epithelium.

between blinks will help you look straight with the eye that is being treated.

Tell your surgeon if you feel faint or sweaty during the procedure. Although rare, it is possible to faint in the middle of a procedure. In most cases this will only delay the treatment and will not cause any serious complications. Communicating with your surgeon will allow your surgeon and staff to take measures to make you more comfortable and in most cases avoid fainting.

After the epithelium is removed the laser will be aligned. You will be instructed to look at the target light. The target light will be blurry and may look like it is moving from your heart beat and breathing. It may help to think about looking through the light as if you are looking at the ceiling to avoid trying to follow the light around. Many lasers have an eye tracker which will follow small movements of the eye called saccades. The laser will stop firing if you look away from the target. The surgeon will realign the laser and resume. In general this will not affect the laser treatment. However, repeatedly looking away will prolong the laser treatment and may increase the chance of retreatment.

As it fires, the laser will make a loud snapping noise like a bug zapper. The sound will be accompanied by a smell like burnt hair or branding that is the result of the particles released as the corneal tissue is ablated (evaporated) by the laser. It is not possible to completely remove this smell. When the laser treatment is complete drops are placed along with a bandage contact lens to protect the cornea as it is healing.

Healing

Just like with PRK the bandage contact lens will stay in place for three or four days following Epi-LASIK. Most people find that discomfort and vision will get worse over the first two days. Often the discomfort is mild, with many people describing it like having a contact lens in too long. However, some people become very light sensitive and have significant discomfort. It may be necessary to stay in a dark room for the first few days and take the pain medications that are provided following Epi-LASIK.

After Epi-LASIK spend as much time as possible with the eyes closed for the first three days, and plan to take it very easy for three to four days following Epi-LASIK. Antibiotic and anti-inflammatory drops will be prescribed following surgery. Preservative free artificial tears are recommended for the first few days after Epi-LASIK. Preservatives can slow healing or cause irritation. A freezing drop is also provided in most cases. Overuse of the freezing drop can slow healing so should be used sparingly. This drop will give you about twenty minutes of relief which may be enough to get back to sleep. If the contact lens falls out you should replace it with a new lens. You will need to call your surgeon if you can not replace the lens yourself.

It is possible that small hemorrhages (small spots of blood) may be present in the conjunctiva overlaying the white part of the eye (sclera). These can result from the suction ring used to stabilize the epikeratome and do not cause any problems. They can take a week or longer to resolve in some cases.

Often your surgeon or staff will check your eyes the day after surgery. This is a safety check to make sure there are no signs of infection or inflammation. It is expected the comfort and vision will worsen over the next two days, and in most cases there will be a check on the third or fourth day after surgery. The contact lenses will be removed on the third day or fourth day in most cases. Differences in healing mean there are a few people who may have the contact in place for a longer period of time.

When the contact lens is removed you may be legal to drive. Legal to drive is a few lines away from 20/20 and driving standards vary between states and provinces. Due to differences in healing some people may not be legal to drive for up to five to seven days following Epi-LASIK, so do not plan to return to work in the first week. Some people might resume modified work at four or five days following surgery but it is less stressful to plan to have a longer time off work following Epi-LASIK. Do not resume driving or other visually demanding activities until you are advised by your surgeon and you feel comfortable with your vision.

Following Epi-LASIK many people have some vision fluctuation for four to eight weeks. A brighter light, more frequent breaks from computer or reading, and limiting night driving may be necessary during this time. Frequent artificial tears may help. Most people find overall sharpness of vision, dry eye symptoms, and night vision will improve over this time. It is important to be patient with your recovery and plan to take breaks or limit night driving if needed. Patience during the first days and weeks following Epi-LASIK is essential. Your eye care provider should be contacted if you have any concerns about your level of vision or other symptoms.

Medicated drops may be recommended for up to six months following surgery to avoid regression (healing back towards your original prescription). Dryness, night vision

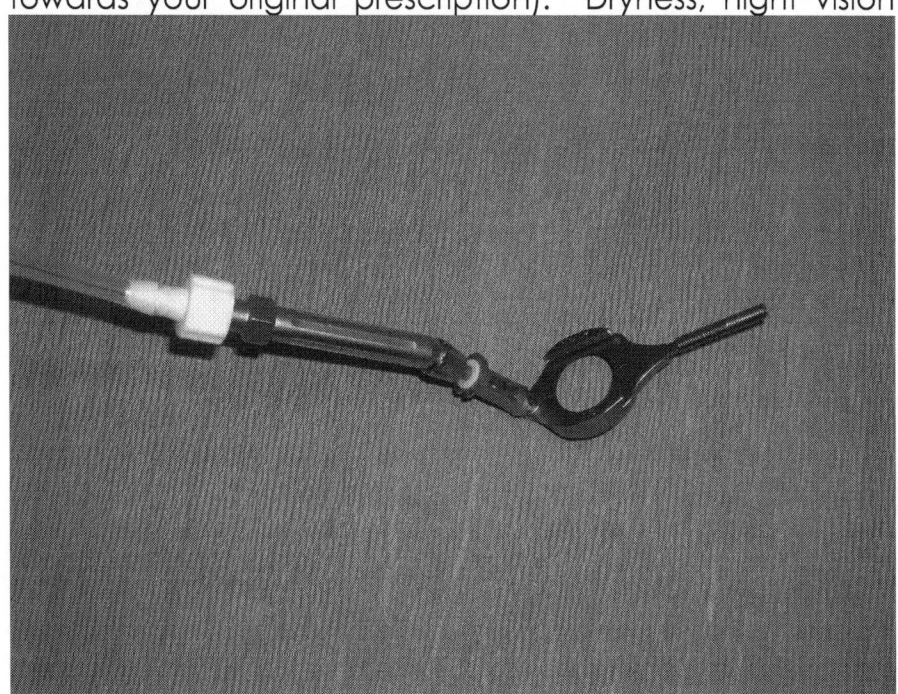

The epikeratome attaches to the suction ring which stabilizes the eye during epithelium removal.

problems, and overall sharpness of vision will usually continue over several weeks to months after surgery.

Post-operative Care

Following uncomplicated Epi-LASIK you will most likely have a check on the first day following surgery and then within a few days after surgery to remove the bandage contact lens. Once the bandage contact lens has been removed and you are in the legal range for driving, there will usually be a post-operative check once a month for up to six months depending on the healing response.

Complications

Epi-LASIK is very safe and has become popular among surgeons over the past few years. The risk of complications during surgery is very low. It is possible that during surgery irregular astigmatism can be created during the epithelial removal step, and loose epithelium outside of the treatment zone can result in delayed healing. Corneal scars may pose a risk for irregularity (also called stromal incursion) at the time of surgery. Map-dot-fingerprint, a corneal dystrophy, may pose a risk for loose epithelium at the time of surgery. A decentration of the laser treatment or other factors could lead to irregularity of the surface of the eye. In most cases this type of irregularity can be corrected with additional surgery.

Intra Operative Epi-LASIK Complications

Stromal incursion: corneal irregularity caused by the Epikeratome at the time of surgery that is more common with history of corneal scar.

Loose epithelium: loose epithelium around the treatment zone at the time of surgery may delay healing. This is more common with some corneal conditions such as map-dot-fingerprint.

Decentration: a very uncommon situation where the treatment zone is not centered over the visual axis.

Chapter 9: Epi-LASIK

Post-operative complications of Epi-LASIK are also uncommon, but again the risk is not zero.

Post Operative Epi-LASIK Complications

Infection: infection might develop within the first few days following surgery. In most cases infection can be treated.

Scar/Haze: with newer lasers it is very uncommon to have significant scar or corneal haze.

Under or overcorrection: a small percentage of people will over or under respond to laser vision correction. Once the correction has stabilized in most cases an enhancement can be done.

Recurrent erosion: in some cases the corneal epithelium develops a weakness following surgery that can result in a spontaneous abrasion. In many cases this can be treated with topical drops.

Regression: in some cases the eye heals back in the direction of the original prescription. This can be treated by a retreatment.

Ectasia: in very rare cases corneal instability can result from laser vision correction surgery.

Dry eye: dry eye is the most common side effect of any laser vision correction surgery.

Night vision changes: although uncommon glare and halo at night may worsen following any type of laser vision correction.

These are the most common possible complications. As with all laser vision correction surgeries many people are more sensitive to irritants in the air such as smoke. This may be permanent and is likely due to the fact that the cornea is more exposed once there are no contact lenses or glasses to protect the cornea. It is not possible to predict all possible complications. The testing done during the laser vision assessment is intended to identify people who may be at high risk for complications of laser vision correction.

Most complications of Epi-LASIK will either resolve over time or may be treated with medications or further surgery. In some cases corrective lenses may be needed to improve vision. In rare cases there may be complications following Epi-LASIK that may lead to a loss of vision that can not be treated.

Enhancement (retreatment) after Epi-LASIK

Epi-LASIK involves the treatment of the corneal surface which is living tissue and so can heal and respond differently in different individuals. A small percentage of people will need a second treatment, known as an enhancement or retreatment, for their best vision. In all cases the correction needs to stabilize before additional surgery can be done. This may take six months or longer in some cases. A few people may have a need for a corrective lens for driving while they are waiting for enhancement.

Retreatment following Epi-LASIK will be either alcohol assisted PRK or may be PRK with a brush. Due to the fact the corneal surface has been altered it is not possible to use the Epi-keratome for retreatments. The majority of time the amount of residual correction is low enough or affects only one eye so it may be possible to drive and do usual activities without corrective lenses while waiting for the cornea to stabilize.

Chapter 9: Epi-LASIK

Reasons for Retreatment after Epi-LASIK

Regression: healing back towards the original correction.

Under-response: a residual amount of correction can remain if the corneal tissue does not respond as expected to the laser treatment.

Over-correction: the intended correction can result in an over-correction if the cornea responds more than anticipated to the laser treatment.

Irregular astigmatism/ scarring/haze: with newer lasers it is uncommon to have significant haze, scarring, or corneal irregularities after PRK.

Regression is healing which causes the eye to shift back towards the original prescription. Regression is more common in higher corrections and in far-sighted corrections. A mild steroid drop is usually recommended for three to six months following Epi-LASIK to reduce the chance of regression. A tapering schedule such as four drops per day for the first month then three drops per day for the second month and so on is the most common recommendation. The schedule might be modified in order to slow healing further or in some cases reduced more quickly to encourage more rapid healing. If regression occurs you will have to wait up to six months or longer for the correction to stabilize before considering an enhancement. While on steroid eye drops the pressure will be monitored periodically as there are some individuals who may develop elevated eye pressure due to steroid drops.

If the amount of tissue removed with the excimer laser is less than intended an under-correction or an under-response will result. There are several theoretic reasons for this including corneal hydration and ambient humidity. Laser centers will have their excimer laser in a climate controlled room with a constant temperature and humidity to avoid fluctuations in laser energy that is delivered to the cornea. Surgeons will usually use a standard surgical technique in order to avoid variations in corneal hydration during Epi-LASIK.

Factors such as degree of correction and age will be taken into consideration when entering the laser data in order to compensate for the likelihood of under-response. Mitomycin-C is a medication that may be used at the time of surgery for high corrections to slow healing and prevent regression. In spite of all these measures, there are some people who will under-respond to the treatment. In these cases there will be residual correction measured immediately after surgery. It is still necessary to wait for up to six months before enhancement surgery to make sure the correction is stable.

The same factors described above can lead to an over-correction which is sometimes called an over-response. When over-correction happens the measured prescription will be opposite the original correction. If an over correction occurs you may have been near-sighted (myopic) before surgery and then far-sighted (hyperopic) immediately following surgery. Over-correction of far-sightedness will result in a near-sighted prescription immediately following Epi-LASIK. Your surgeon may modify post-operative drops to encourage faster healing in these cases.

Regression or healing back towards the original correction will lead to self correction of a small over-correction over the weeks and months following surgery in many cases. For Epi-LASIK a mild over-correction is expected in the first several weeks, and the cornea usually settles a little back towards the original prescription. For a significant over-correction it may be necessary to wear reading glasses or distance glasses while waiting for the prescription to stabilize.

Depending on how high the starting prescription is, the enhancement rates may range from five to fifteen percent. The higher the prescription the more likely you might need a second treatment for your best vision. It is very uncommon to do more than one enhancement, although in rare cases it may be necessary. Repeated enhancements are usually not recommended.

If the prescription is unstable there may be other factors such as cataracts or diabetes that are having an effect on the eye. There may be some cases when your surgeon may recommend against any further surgery, and you may be back into glasses or contact lenses. Although this is uncommon you and your surgeon need to weigh the risks and benefits of each repeat surgery before deciding to proceed.

For haze, scarring, or irregular astigmatism following Epi-LASIK surgery more complex retreatments may be needed. A smoothing treatment can sometimes be done with the laser called phototherapeutic keratectomy or PTK. If you need PTK your surgeon should discuss the treatment plan and expectations with you before retreatment.

Summary

Epi-LASIK is an excellent option for most people who qualify for laser vision correction. It is a lower risk compared to flap procedures due to the simplicity of this technique, but a slightly higher risk than PRK due to the use of the epikeratome. The risk is never zero. Epi-LASIK usually provides a more rapid return to usual activities compared to PRK. For thinner corneas, surface treatments such as PRK or Epi-LASIK may be the only option for laser vision correction. Discuss your options with your surgeon, and be sure to have all your questions answered before deciding if Epi-LASIK is a good option for you.

CHAPTER 10: LASIK

LASIK has been performed in North America since Dr. Pallikaris introduced it in 1992. LASIK was a combination of older lamellar corneal flap techniques combined with the excimer laser. Some have called it "flap and zap". It quickly became popular in the late 1990's as it offered more rapid recovery of vision and less discomfort compared to PRK. LASIK does carry a higher risk than no-flap procedures (PRK and Epi-LASIK) due to the fact that it does affect the cornea to a deeper level and creating a flap is a more complex technique.

How is LASIK done?

As with other types of laser vision correction treatments, the eye is frozen with drops. A lid holder (speculum) is placed on the eye to hold the lids open, and the speculum may give you a pinching or pulling sensation as you blink since the lids are not frozen. The other eye may be covered with a patch. A sedative is usually offered, and it is a good idea to take it. The sedative will not make you sleepy, but it help the procedure go more smoothly.

A microkeratome is used to create the flap. The microkeratome uses a suction ring to stabilize the eye. During this step in the procedure you will feel pressure and the vision will dim out for about thirty seconds. You may feel an additional pinching on the lid while the flap is created and there will be a buzzing sensation during this time. Once the pressure is released the vision returns but will be blurry.

If you feel unwell it is important to tell your surgeon. In the rare case that someone faints, it will not result usually any problems but can delay the surgery. Fainting can be avoided by letting your surgeon know you don't feel well. A cold cloth on your forehead, a break, a drink some juice or water, or a simple repositioning can be helpful in many cases. Putting a pillow under the knees to help

Laser Vision Correction

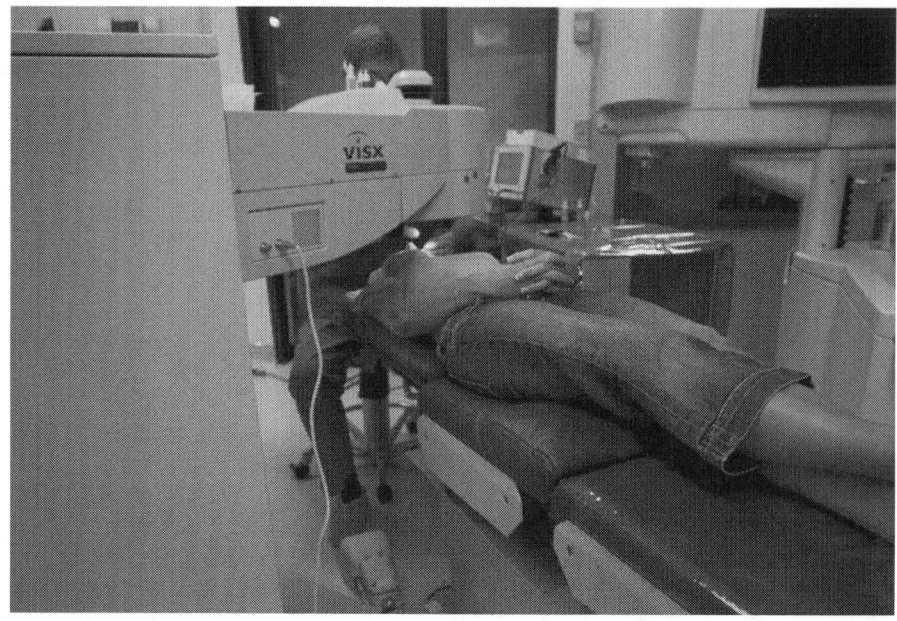

your back or other measures can help. The more comfortable you are the more quickly the procedure will be completed.

Once the corneal flap is lifted, the laser will be aligned. You will be instructed to look at the target light. The target light will look blurry and will look like it is moving from your heart-beat and breathing. It may help to look through the light as if you are looking at the ceiling to avoid trying to follow the light around. Looking away from the target will cause the laser to stop. The surgeon will realign the laser and continue the treatment. Looking away repeatedly could lead to a higher chance of needing a retreatment. Many lasers have an eye tracker that will follow saccades which are small movements of the eye.

As it fires the laser makes a loud snapping noise like a bug zapper. This is accompanied by a smell like burnt hair (or branding) which is the result of the particles released as the corneal tissue is ablated (evaporated) by the excimer laser. It is not possible to eliminate the smell completely, even with a suction tube.

When the laser is complete the flap is repositioned. Antibiotics and anti-inflammatory drops are instilled. In some cases protective bubbles with adhesives will be applied to protect the flaps.

Healing

Most people will find their vision to be very blurry for the first twenty-four hours following LASIK. In many cases the eyes may sting or burn or it may feel like something is in the eye. In many cases the two eyes will feel different or the vision may clear faster in one eye than the other. You may notice a small hemorrhage or spot of blood in the conjunctiva which lines the whites of the eye (sclera). These sometimes result from the suction ring used during surgery and do not cause any problems. They may take one or two weeks to clear.

Many people will be legal to drive on the first day, however legal to drive may not be 20/20. It may be necessary to limit night driving for a period of time. Some people will continue to experience some dryness or irritation for days to weeks.

Fluctuations in vision, sharpness of vision, dry eye, and night vision will continue to improve over the first few months. Frequent artificial tears may be helpful during this time. Modification of work, hobbies, and driving habits may be helpful during this time. If you plan for this, you will experience less stress during the first weeks following surgery. If you have any concerns you during your healing you should discuss it with your surgeon.

Post-operative Care

In an uncomplicated LASIK case it is likely that you will have a post operative check within the first few days following surgery. Depending on the vision and healing the next visit may be one to three months post-operatively.

Complications

LASIK has been performed in North America for over fifteen years. While the majority of patients do well there are some risks.

Intra-Operative Complications

Incomplete flap:	there are a number of reasons that an incomplete flap may be created; it is possible a new flap could be created at a future time.
Buttonhole:	in some cases the center of the flap is very thin. In many cases a new flap could be created at a future time.
Thin flap:	If the flap is extremely thin the surgeon may choose to reposition the flap and consider treatment at a later date.
Decentration:	decentration of the laser treatment is very unlikely; many lasers have an eye tracker which helps to avoid this complication.
Loose epithelium:	in some cases the surface epithelium will be loose on the surface of the flap or around the edge of the flap. This may delay healing.

Although uncommon, there are complications that can occur in the days or weeks following LASIK.

Chapter 10: LASIK

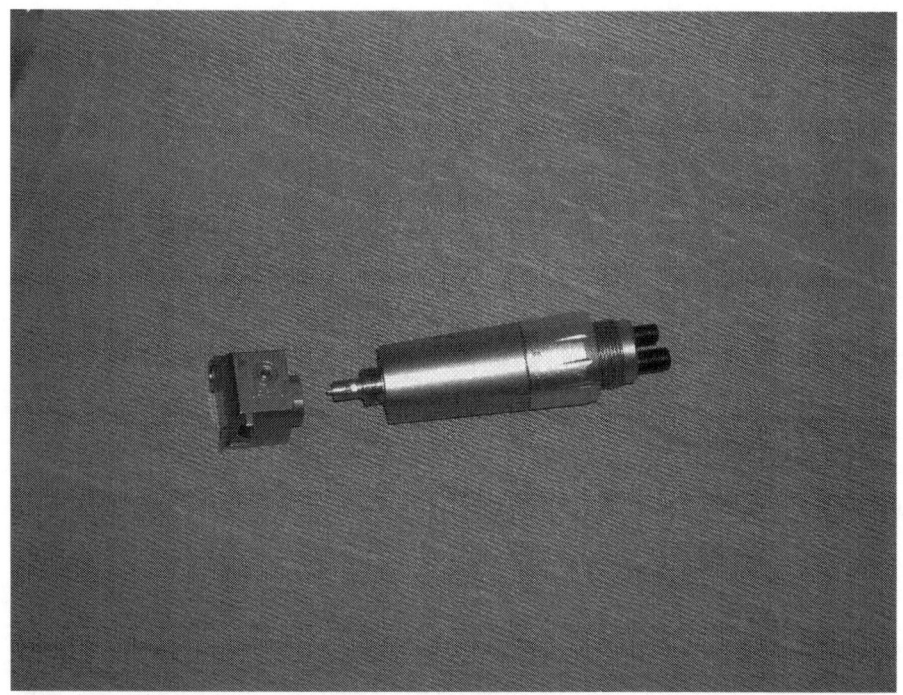

The microkeratome consists of a motor housed in a handpiece which drives the microkeratome head that contains an oscillating blade to cut a precise corneal flap during LASIK surgery.

Post Operative LASIK Complications

Infection: it is possible that infection might develop within the first few days following surgery. In most cases infection can be treated.

Scar/haze: with newer lasers it is very uncommon to have significant scar or corneal haze.

Diffuse lamellar keratitis (DLK): also called "Sands of Saraha" due to the appearance of inflammation at the flap interface; may be triggered by injury or a reaction to substances at the time of surgery; can be treated in most cases.

Under or overcorrection: a small percentage of people will over or under respond to laser vision correction; once the correction has stabilized in most cases an enhancement can be done.

Epithelial ingrowth: in some cases the corneal epithelium will grow under the LASIK flap; this is more common with enhancements.

Regression: in some cases the eye heals back in the direction of the original prescription. This can be treated by a retreatment.

Ectasia: in very rare cases corneal instability can result from laser vision correction surgery.

Flap dislocation: it is possible to shift or damage the flap days, months, or years post surgery; usually from direct corneal injury; usually flap can be repositioned.

Dry eye: dry eye is the most common side effect of any laser vision correction.

Night vision changes: although uncommon glare and halo at night may worsen following any type of laser vision correction.

The list above contains the most common possible complications. It is not possible to predict all possible complications, but pre-operative testing is intended to identify people who may be at high risk for complications of laser vision correction.

Ectasia is a rare but feared complication which is more common following LASIK than with surface no-flap treat-

Chapter 10: LASIK

ments such as PRK or Epi-LASIK. The risk of ectasia even with no-flap procedures is never zero. There are several factors the surgeon will consider before allowing you to undergo LASIK. Many surgeons have a minimum total corneal thickness they require before considering performing laser vision correction. Most surgeons in North America will use 250 microns as their minimum residual bed thickness in order to avoid over thinning of the cornea which may be associated with ectasia, and there has been some discussion as to whether the minimum should be 300 microns. The residual bed is calculated as the total corneal thickness minus the LASIK flap thickness and minus the amount of tissue to be removed by the laser. For thinner corneas or higher corrections a no-flap treatment may be recommended. Other risk factors for ectasia may include corneal mapping abnormalities, very steep corneas, family history of keratoconus, and unstable refraction with increasing astigmatism. Ectasia appears to be due to multiple factors and residual bed thickness is just one of many possible risk factors.

There is a newer LASIK technique called Sub-Bowman's Keratomelieusis (SBK). SBK involves the use of a microkeratome that is designed to create a very thin flap which is on par with the Intra-LASIK flap created by the femtosecond laser. The theory is that the thinner the flap, the less the biomechanical weakening of the cornea, and the less the risk of ectasia. Although the flap does not leave the eye, once it is created it no longer provides the same structural support to the cornea. The flap is a permanent alteration of the corneal structure. It is possible to lift some flaps for retreatments even years later while is some cases the flap is too adherent to lift after one or two years. This fact demonstrates that the healing of the flap is variable between individuals.

In most cases complications of laser vision correction will either resolve over time (in some cases many months) or may be treated with medications or further surgery. In some cases corrective lenses may be needed to improve vision. In rare cases there may be complications following LASIK that may lead to a loss of vision that can not be treated.

Enhancement (retreatment) after LASIK

LASIK involves the treatment of the corneal surface. The cornea is living tissue and so can heal and respond differently in different individuals. A small percentage of people will need a second treatment, known as an enhancement, for their best vision. In all cases the correction needs to stabilize before additional surgery can be done. This may take six months or longer in some cases. A few people may have a need for a corrective lens for driving while they are waiting for enhancement. For many people the amount of residual correction is low or affects only one eye so they may be able to drive and do usual activities without corrective lenses while waiting for the cornea to stabilize.

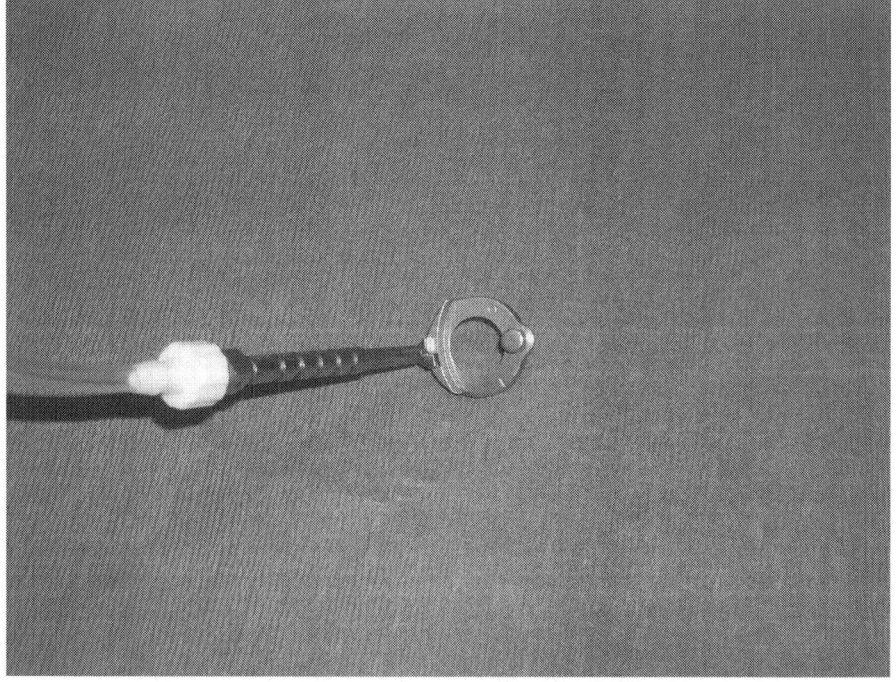

The microkeratome attaches to a suction ring which stabilizes the eye during the creation of the LASIK flap.

Retreatment following LASIK involves lifting the flap, placing the laser treatment, and replacing the flap. Lifting the flap can be done in some cases up to ten years following primary surgery. There are some cases where the flap is too adherent and consideration must be made as to if there is enough residual correction to warrant cutting a new flap. There are some specific situations in which a surface PRK or PTK treatment may be recommended following LASIK surgery.

Reasons for Retreatment after LASIK

Regression:	healing back towards the original correction.
Under-response:	a residual amount of correction can remain if the corneal tissue does not respond as expected to the laser treatment.
Over-correction:	the intended correction can result in an over-correction if the cornea responds more than anticipated to the laser treatment.
Irregular astigmatism/ scarring/haze:	it is uncommon to have significant haze, scarring, or corneal irregularities after LASIK.

Regression is more common in higher corrections and in far-sighted corrections. For higher corrections a special topical medication called mitomycin-C is sometimes used at the time of surgery to slow healing and prevent regression. If regression occurs you may have to wait up to six months or longer for the correction to stabilize before considering an enhancement.

In cases where the amount of tissue removed with the excimer laser is less than intended an under-correction or an under-response may occur. There are several theoretic reasons for this including corneal hydration and ambient humidity. Laser centers will have their excimer laser in a climate controlled room with a constant temperature and humidity to avoid fluctuations in laser energy that is delivered to the cornea. Surgeons will usually use a standard surgical technique in order to avoid variations in corneal hydration during LASIK. In some cases the correction data is adjusted based on factors such as degree of correction and age in order to compensate for the likelihood of under-response in certain cases.

In spite of all these measures there are some people who will under-respond to the treatment. In these cases there will be residual correction measured immediately after surgery. It is still necessary to wait for up to six months before enhancement surgery to make sure the correction is stable.

Similar to under-correction, the same factors described above can lead to an over-correction which is sometimes called an over-response. When over-correction occurs the measured prescription will be opposite the original correction. With an over-correction you may have been near-sighted (myopic) before surgery and then far-sighted (hyperopic) immediately following surgery. Alternatively if you were far-sighted, you may be near-sighted immediately following LASIK. Regression or healing back towards the original correction may lead to self correction of a small over-correction over the weeks and months following surgery. A significant over-correction may result in the need to wear reading glasses or distance glasses while waiting for the prescription to stabilize.

There is a five to fifteen percent chance of enhancement depending on the magnitude of the starting prescription. The higher the prescription the more likely you might need a second treatment for your best vision. It is very uncommon to do more than one enhancement, although in rare cases it may be necessary. Repeated enhancements are usually not recommended. If the prescription is unstable there may be other factors such as cataracts or diabetes that are having an effect on the eye. There may be some cases when your surgeon may recommend against any further surgery and you may be back into glasses or contact lenses. Although this is uncommon you and your surgeon need to weigh the risks and benefits of each repeat surgery before deciding to proceed.

More complicated treatments may be needed for haze, scarring, or irregular astigmatism. In these cases a smoothing treatment can sometimes be done with the laser called phototherapeutic keratectomy or PTK. If you need PTK your surgeon should discuss the treatment plan and expectations with you before retreatment.

Summary

LASIK is a common choice for many people who qualify for laser vision correction. This technique has been in use for over a decade and has good long term results and stability. If you have thin corneas or high risk work or hobbies then a no-flap treatment may be recommended as the best alternative. You should discuss your options with your surgeon and be sure to have all your questions answered before deciding if LASIK is a good option for you.

CHAPTER 11: INTRA-LASIK

Dr. Arturo Chayet is credited with the idea of Intra-LASIK. Intra-LASIK uses the ultra fast femtosecond laser to create a thin corneal flap. The advantages of Intra-LASIK over LASIK are that the flap can be made thinner and is felt to be more uniform than flaps created by a microkeratome. The first Intra-LASIK was performed in 2000.

How is Intra-LASIK done?

The eye is frozen with drops, and a lid holder (speculum) is placed on the eye to hold the lids open. Since the lids are not frozen, the speculum may give you a pinching or pulling sensation as you blink. The other eye may be covered with a patch. A sedative will be recommended. The sedative will not make you sleepy, but it help the procedure go more smoothly.

The femtosecond laser is used to create the flap. This laser uses a device called a cone to deliver the energy to the cornea. A suction ring is placed to stabilize the eye which fits the cone. The cone is pressed onto your cornea for about thirty seconds. During this time your vision will dim or black out, and you will feel pressure. In some cases you may feel a pinching or pressing on the lids. The femtosecond laser is quiet. Once the pressure is released your vision will return but it will be blurry.

Be sure to tell your surgeon if you feel faint. Fainting is uncommon and will not usually result any problems other than delaying the surgery. It can usually be avoided by speaking up so the staff can take a few moments if you are feeling unwell to put a cold cloth on your forehead, let you take a break, or drink some juice or water. Putting a pillow under the knees to help your back or other measures will often help. The more comfortable you are the more quickly the procedure will be completed.

You will be reclining on your back during the procedure. Once the femtosecond laser flap creation is complete, your chair will be rotated to position you under the excimer laser. The corneal flap will be lifted, and the excimer laser will be aligned. You will be instructed to look at the target light.

The target light will look blurry and will look like it is moving from your heart-beat and breathing. It may help to look through the light as if you are looking at the ceiling to avoid trying to follow the light around. Many lasers have an eye tracker which will follow saccades which are small movements of the eye. If you look away, the laser will be stopped and then realigned. This does not usually cause any problems, but if you look away repeatedly it may prolong treatment which can result in higher likelihood of retreatment.

You will hear a snapping noise like a bug zapper and smell an odor like burnt hair or branding as the excimer laser fires. The smell is the result of the particles released as the corneal tissue is ablated (evaporated) by the excimer laser. Unfortunately it is not possible to eliminate the smell completely, even with a suction tube.

When the laser is complete the flap is repositioned. Antibiotics and anti-inflammatory drops are instilled. In some cases protective bubbles with adhesives will be applied to protect the flaps.

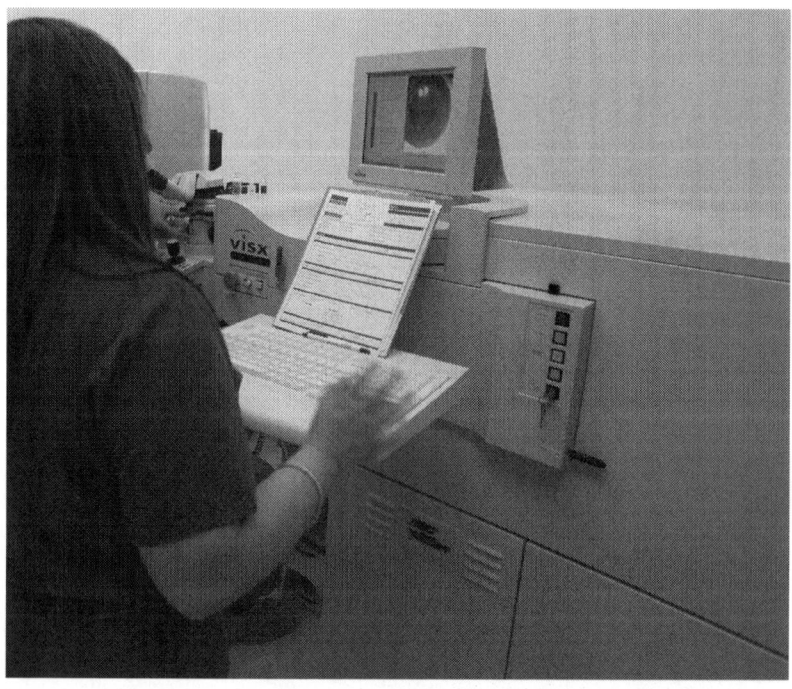

Healing

Most people will find their vision to be very blurry until the next day following Intra-LASIK. In some cases a portion of the cornea may look white temporarily. This is due to gas bubbles trapped in the cornea and should resolve within minutes to hours. This is called an opaque bubble layer (OBL). In many cases the eyes may sting or burn or it may feel like something is in the eye. In many cases the two eyes may feel different or the vision may clear faster in one eye than the other. In some cases small hemorrhages will be visible on the white part of the eye (conjunctiva on top of the sclera). These hemorrhages will resolve in a week to two weeks.

Many people will be legal to drive on the first day, however legal to drive may not be 20/20. It may be necessary to limit night driving for a period of time. Some people will continue to experience some dryness or irritation for days to weeks. Fluctuations in vision, sharpness of vision, dry eye, and night vision will continue to improve over the first few months. Frequent artificial tears may be helpful. Modification of work, hobbies, and driving habits may also be helpful during this time. You can reduce your stress by planning for these side effects during the first several weeks following surgery.

In rare cases some patients may develop significant light sensitivity called photophobia. This will generally respond to treatment with steroid eye drops over several days to a few weeks.

It is likely that any post-operative dryness, night vision problems, and overall sharpness of vision will continue to improve over several weeks to months after surgery. If you have any concerns you during your healing you should discuss it with your surgeon.

Post-operative Care

In an uncomplicated Intra-LASIK case it is likely that you will have a post operative check within the first few days following surgery. Depending on the vision and healing the next visit may be one to three months post-operatively.

Complications

Intra-LASIK has gained in popularity over the past few years. The risks of creating a flap with the femtosecond laser are felt to be less than creating the flap with the microkeratome. While the majority of patients do well, there are some risks.

Intra-Operative Complications

Incomplete flap:	there are a number of reasons that an incomplete flap may be created; it is possible a new flap could be created within a short time.
Buttonhole:	in some cases the center of the flap is very thin. This will be less likely to occur with Intra-LASIK.
Thin flap:	If the flap is extremely thin the surgeon may choose to reposition the flap and consider treatment at a later date.
Decentration:	decentration of the laser treatment is very unlikely; many lasers have an eye tracker which helps to avoid this complication.
Loose epithelium:	in some cases the surface epithelium will be loose on the surface of the flap or around the edge of the flap. This may delay healing.
Opaque bubble layer (OBL):	it is possible for the gas generated by femtosecond laser treatment to become trapped in the cornea and create a white opaque layer. In some cases the excimer treatment must be delayed to let this clear.

Chapter 11: Intra-LASIK

Anterior chamber gas bubble: it is possible for the gas generated during Intra-LASIK to enter the eye. In some cases the excimer treatment must be delayed until this clears.

Although uncommon, there are also complications that can occur in the days or weeks following Intra-LASIK.

Post Operative Intra-LASIK Complications

Infection: it is possible that infection might develop within the first few days following surgery. In most cases infection can be treated.

Scar/haze: with newer lasers it is very uncommon to have significant scar or corneal haze.

Photosensitivity: some patients will experience significant sensitivity to light following Intra-LASIK; this can be treated with steroid drops for days to in some cases a few weeks.

Diffuse lamellar keratitis (DLK): also called "Sands of Saraha" due to the appearance of inflammation at the flap interface; may be triggered by injury or a reaction to substances at the time of surgery; can be treated in most cases.

Under or overcorrection: a small percentage of people will over or under respond to laser vision correction; once the correction has stabilized in most cases an enhancement can be done.

Epithelial ingrowth:	in some cases the corneal epithelium will grow under the LASIK flap; this is more common with enhancements.
Regression:	in some cases the eye heals back in the direction of the original prescription. This can be treated by a retreatment.
Ectasia:	in very rare cases corneal instability can result from laser vision correction surgery.
Flap dislocation:	it is possible to shift or damage the flap days, months, or years post surgery; usually from direct corneal injury; usually flap can be repositioned.
Dry eye:	dry eye is the most common side effect of any laser vision correction.
Night vision changes:	although uncommon glare and halo at night may worsen following any type of laser vision correction.

The list above contains the most common possible complications. It is not possible to predict all possible complications, but in the pre-operative testing is intended to identify people who may be at high risk for complications of laser vision correction.

Ectasia is a rare but feared complication which is more common following LASIK than with surface no-flap treatments such as PRK or Epi-LASIK. The technique of Intra-LASIK is relatively new, but theoretically the risk of ectasia with Intra-LASIK may be lower than with LASIK because the flap can be made thinner. However, newer microkeratomes are becoming available which can make very thin LASIK flaps so the difference may not be significant. The risk of ectasia even with no-flap procedures is never zero.

There are several factors the surgeon will consider before allowing you to undergo Intra-LASIK. Many surgeons have a minimum total corneal thickness they require before considering performing laser vision correction. Most surgeons in North America will use 250 microns as their minimum residual bed thickness in order to avoid over thinning of the cornea which may be associated with ectasia. The residual bed is calculated as the total corneal thickness minus the Intra-LASIK flap thickness and minus the amount of tissue to be removed by the laser. For thinner corneas or higher corrections a no-flap treatment may be recommended. Other risk factors for ectasia may include corneal mapping abnormalities, very steep corneas, family history of keratoconus, and unstable refraction with increasing astigmatism. Corneal thickness is one fact among several which have been associated with ectasia.

In most cases complications of laser vision correction will either resolve over time or may be treated with medications or further surgery. In some cases corrective lenses may be needed to improve vision. In rare cases there may be complications following Intra-LASIK that may lead to a loss of vision that may not be treatable.

Enhancement (retreatment) after Intra-LASIK

Because the cornea is living tissue, it can heal and respond differently in different individuals. A small percentage of people will need a second treatment, known as an enhancement, for their best vision. In all cases the correction needs to stabilize before additional surgery can be done. This may take six months or longer in some cases. A few people may have a need for a corrective lens for driving while they are waiting for enhancement. For many people the amount of residual correction is low enough or affects only one eye so they may be able to drive and do usual activities without corrective lenses while waiting for the cornea to stabilize.

Retreatments following Intra-LASIK involve lifting the corneal flap, ablating the bed to achieve the additional correction, and then replacing the flap. The risks of lifting the flap are less than the risk of creating a new flap. The recovery following enhancement will be similar to the recovery following a primary Intra-LASIK.

Reasons for Retreatment after Intra-LASIK

Regression: healing back towards the original correction.

Under-response: a residual amount of correction can remain if the corneal tissue does not respond as expected to the laser treatment.

Over-correction: the intended correction can result in an over-correction if the cornea responds more than anticipated to the laser treatment.

Irregular astigmatism/ scarring/haze: it is uncommon to have significant haze, scarring, or corneal irregularities after Intra-LASIK.

When the eye heals back towards the original prescription it is called regression. This is more common in higher corrections and in far-sighted corrections. Topical mitomycin-C is sometimes used at the time of surgery to slow healing and prevent regression. You may have to wait up to six months or longer for the correction to stabilize before considering an enhancement.

Sometimes the amount of tissue removed with the excimer laser might be less than intended. This is known as an under-correction or an under-response. There are several theoretic reasons for this including corneal hydration

Chapter 11: Intra-LASIK

and ambient humidity. Laser centers will have their excimer laser in a climate controlled room with a constant temperature and humidity to avoid fluctuations in laser energy that is delivered to the cornea. Surgeons will usually use a standard surgical technique in order to avoid variations in corneal hydration during LASIK. In some cases the correction data is altered based on factors such as degree of correction and age in order to compensate for the likelihood of under-response in certain cases.

Some people will under-respond to the treatment in spite of all these precautions. In these cases there will be residual correction measured immediately after surgery. It is still necessary to wait for up to six months before enhancement surgery to make sure the correction is stable.

The same factors described above can lead to an over-correction which is sometimes called an over-response. Over-correction occurs when the measured prescription is opposite the original correction such that you may have been near-sighted (myopic) before surgery and then far-sighted (hyperopic) immediately following surgery. If you were far-sighted to start with, you may be near-sighted immediately following LASIK if there is an over-correction. Healing back towards the original correction, called regression, may lead to self correction of a small over-correction over the weeks and months following surgery. A significant over-correction may result in the need to wear reading glasses or distance glasses while waiting for the prescription to stabilize.

The higher the prescription the more likely you might need a second treatment for your best vision. Retreatment rates vary from five to fifteen percent depending on the starting prescription. In rare cases it may be necessary to do more than one enhancement. Repeated enhancements are usually not recommended. An unstable refraction may be caused by other factors such as cataracts or diabetes that are having an effect on the eye. In some cases your surgeon may recommend against any further surgery, and you may be back into glasses or contact lenses. You and your surgeon need to weigh the risks and benefits of each repeat surgery before deciding to proceed.

More complicated treatments may be needed for haze, scarring, or irregular astigmatism. In these cases a smoothing treatment can sometimes be done with the laser called phototherapeutic keratectomy or PTK. If you are needing PTK your surgeon should discuss the treatment plan and expectations with you before retreatment.

Summary

Intra-LASIK is becoming a more common choice for many people who qualify for laser vision correction. This technique is relatively new but has shown good results and may be safer than LASIK. Those with thin corneas may still be recommended to undergo a no-flap treatment. You should discuss your options with your surgeon and be sure to have all your questions answered before deciding if Intra-LASIK is a good choice for you.

CHAPTER 12: LASER TYPES

There are several different lasers that are used in eye surgery. Each laser has specific applications.

Ophthalmic Lasers

Excimer laser: gases such as Argon and Fluoride are used to create "excited dimers". Excimer lasers produce light with 193 nm ultraviolet wavelength which is ideal for corneal laser vision correction.

Femtosecond laser: this laser uses an ultrafast infrared pulse at 1053nm to create precise confluent gas bubbles which are used to create the Intra-LASIK flap.

Holmium Laser: this laser is used to apply heat to precise spots on the cornea for the treatment of hyperopia. This is called laser thermokeratoplasty (LTK).

YAG Laser: this is a solid state laser used to treat secondary cataracts (posterior capsular fibrosis) following cataract surgery, treatment of narrow angle glaucoma with peripheral iridotomies, and selective laser trabeculoplasty (SLT) for certain types of glaucoma.

Argon laser: the argon laser is frequently used for treatment of retinal disorders and can also be used for peripheral iridotomy and argon laser trabeculoplasty (ALT) for treatment of some types of glaucoma.

Excimer Lasers

PRK, Epi-LASIK, LASIK, and Intra-LASIK treatments all utilize the excimer laser to ablate the corneal tissue to precisely correct nearsightedness, farsightedness, and astigmatism. Newer excimer lasers have the capacity to fine tune the correction by treating small irregularities called higher order aberrations.

FDA Approved Excimer Lasers

MEL 80:	Carl Zeiss
Wavelight Allegretto:	Alcon Laboratories
Bausch & Lomb Technolas 217A & 217z:	Technolas GMBH Perfect Vision
VISX Star S4 IR:	Abbott Medical Optics
LASERSCAN LSX:	Lasersight Technologies
EC-5000:	Nidek Inc.
LADARVISION:	Alcon Laboratories

Excimer lasers can be divided into three categories: scanning slit, scanning spot, and broad beam. These designations refer to the pattern of the beam as it exits the laser. With newer lasers the broad beam and scanning slit patterns can be further modified by internal apertures to create more complex patterns such as variable spot size. Some lasers employ variable repetition rate to reduce heat generation which is theorized to reduce the risk of haze.

Wavefront laser treatments involve the measurement of what is called higher order aberrations of an individual's eye and then using those measurements to create a unique treatment plan that is used by the excimer laser to treat the cornea. A wavefront treatment is a tailored treatment

Chapter 12: Laser Types

based on the individual variations of an eye. The Alcon LADARVision, VISX S4 by AMO, and the Baush &Lomb Technolas 217z zyoptics platforms can all do wavefront treatments. The Wavelight Allegretto uses a wavefront optimized system. Some lasers also have the capacity for iris recognition with cyclotorsion adjustment. Cyclotorsion is the rotation of the eye when laying flat. The eye can rotate up to fifteen degrees, but more often may rotate less than five degrees between the upright and supine (laying on your back) positions. It is helpful to adjust for this rotation when undertaking a complex wavefront treatment on the cornea. Wavefront treatments may offer better visual results.

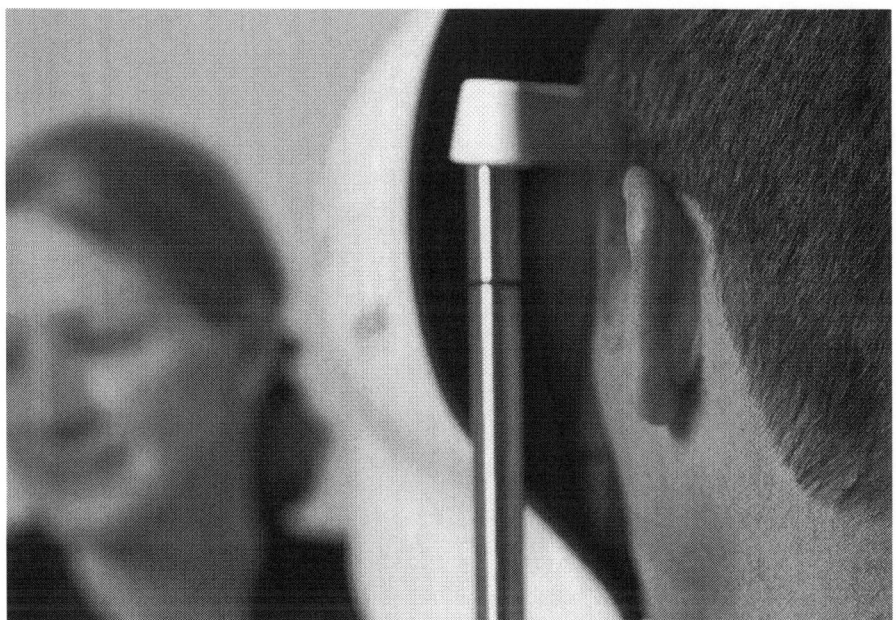

Wavefront mapping is used to measure the individual higher order aberrations. This information is used to create the treatment pattern for use in customized wavefront excimer laser treatments. Photo by Dave Best.

Some laser treatments will create an aspheric shape which mimics the natural shape of the cornea. There is some evidence to suggest that this aspheric shape may optimize results. An aspheric correction is not a wavefront correction.

Excimer lasers may have differences in optical zones and transition zones. The optical zone is the central treatment zone where the majority of the correction is achieved. The transition zone is also sometimes called the blend zone. This blend zone is important in avoiding a sharp transition between the central optical zone and the remaining cornea outside of the treatment zone which is naturally flatter. There has been discussion in the past about the optical zone and transition zone sizes and possible night vision problems. For newer lasers these zones are large enough that it is unusual to have problems with glare and halo following laser vision correction. Pupil size, which has also been discussed in past, has never been definitively correlated with an increased incidence of night vision difficulties.

It is difficult to compare results between lasers since there are different lasers, different surgeons, and different procedures. There have been no large scale studies to prove that one system is better than another. It may be helpful to know what laser will be used in your procedure and to speak to your surgeon about the benefits of that particular laser system. The excimer laser type is one of many factors that must be considered when deciding whether to have laser vision correction, what procedure to have, and what center to choose.

Femtosecond Laser

The femtosecond laser is used in Intra-LASIK. Intra-LASIK is used to designate the use of the femtosecond laser in the creation of a flap for the purpose of laser vision correction. This term is used due to the fact that Intralase® was the first system approved. In addition to the Intralase®, the Da Vinci, Femtec, Femto LDV, Visumax, and Lensx 550 have been approved by the FDA.

There is consensus among surgeons who use the femtosecond laser to create Intra-LASIK flaps that it is safer than the microkeratomes used for LASIK. Some surgeons call Intra-LASIK "all laser LASIK". Femtosecond laser technology is relatively new and there are fewer devices in current use as compared to the number of excimer laser systems. As this technology evolves the consumer will likely have more choices with respect to specific femtosecond laser systems.

Femtosecond lasers are also promising in other types of corneal surgery. If you are considering Intra-LASIK it may be helpful for you to discuss with your surgeon any questions you may have about the technology at that specific center.

Holmium Laser

This laser uses infrared energy to create heat which shrinks precise spots on the cornea in a process called laser thermokeratoplasty. This method of hyperopia treatment is not as popular as excimer laser treatments but is suitable for lower hyperopes. The effect of the holmium laser may wear off over time, and the treatment may need to be repeated.

YAG & Argon Lasers

These lasers are not used to do laser vision correction. For the implantable contact lens a pre-treatment with a YAG iridotomy is necessary to reduce the possibility of increased intraocular pressure.

Argon lasers are more commonly used for retinal applications such as the treatment of diabetic retinopathy.

Summary

It is important to consider all the factors including laser type, surgeon, procedure type, and location when deciding where to have laser vision correction.

CHAPTER 13: ALTERNATE (NON-LASER) VISION CORRECTION OPTIONS

Even if you are a candidate for laser vision correction it may be helpful to know what other options may be available.

Non-Laser Vision Correction

Corrective lenses (glasses & contacts):	some people choose to stay with glasses or contact lenses.
Phakic-IOL/implantable contact lens (ICL):	some people who may not qualify for laser vision correction might qualify for a lens which is implanted in the front of the eye.
Refractive lensectomy:	for this treatment the lens of the eye is removed and replaced with a lens implant similar to how cataract surgery is done.
Thermokeratoplasty:	this is a technique for treating farsighted corrections. Laser (LTK) or radiofrequency (CTK) energy is used to shrink precise spots on the cornea.
Astigmatic keratotomy:	relaxing incision on the cornea to treat astigmatism. This technique is most often done in combination with cataract surgery.

Radial keratotomy (RK): RK involves radial corneal relaxing incisions used to treat nearsightedness. RK would not be done routinely in North America as it is not as precise or stable as laser vision correction.

Corrective Lenses

Many people who are candidates for laser vision correction may choose to stay in glasses or contact lenses in order to avoid the small but real risk of laser vision correction. Some people may be motivated to seek laser vision correction due to discomfort in contact lenses. There are many options for eye glasses and contact lenses. If you are not a candidate for vision correction surgery, working with your eye care provider may help you to stay in contacts at least part time.

Contact lenses may pose a risk for significant corneal infection if they are worn too much. Other risk factors include sleeping in contacts or going in swimming pools, freshwater, or hot-tubs with your contacts in. If you choose to stay in contacts or need to stay in contacts because you are not a candidate for laser vision correction, make sure you follow the recommendations of your eyecare provider in order to avoid a serious corneal infection.

If you are a candidate for laser vision correction and currently have discomfort with contact lenses, this may indicate you are at higher risk for significant permanent dry eye following treatment. It is helpful to treat any underlying conditions which may be causing this discomfort, such as dry eye, blepharitis, or allergies, prior to undergoing laser vision correction.

Phakic IOL

The phakic IOL is an intraocular lens implant that is placed in front of the lens of the eye. Some people who

Chapter 13: Alternate (non-laser) Vision Correction Options

are not candidates for corneal laser surgery may qualify for this option. The Staar Lens is called the ICL® which stands for Implantable Contact Lens. This is a commonly used lens in North America.

The phakic IOL is placed inside the eye and carries a risk of intraocular infection, increased intraocular pressure (glaucoma), and cataract. These risks are low but could result in a need to remove the phakic IOL or a need for cataract surgery. To reduce the chance of increased intraocular pressure tiny holes in the iris are made with a YAG laser prior to implantation of the lens. This is called peripheral iridotomy and is a treatment that is also done for people with a condition called narrow angles.

Phakic IOL may be a good option for some people and can also treat astigmatism if a toric lens is used. Due to this risk of cataract, it may be a better option for patients who are a bit older and already close to needing reading glasses. If it is necessary to do a cataract surgery, reading glasses may be needed afterwards. People with very small anterior chambers (the space between the iris and the cornea) may not qualify for this option. Your eye care provider should be able to either answer your questions or direct you to someone in your area with experience with phakic IOL.

Refractive Lensectomy

This option may be recommended for people over the age of 55 or people who have early lens changes. For refractive lensectomy the lens of the eye is removed and replaced with an intraocular lens implant. This is essentially the same as what is done for cataract surgery except that it is done for people who do not have cataracts to reduce dependence on glasses. This is also called "clear lensectomy" as it removes and replaces a clear lens that does not have a significant cataract.

The reason it may be a better option for older patients is that people in this age range will already need reading glasses or bifocal lenses. Many lens implants will correct for distance only and reading glasses will still be needed or a monovision (one eye left near-sighted for reading) correction can be done. There are new implants with multifocal capabilities, however, they are not widely used for refractive lensectomy at this time. It is quite possible that in the future the multifocal lens implants may be used to correct vision for distance and near for patients in the appropriate age group.

The risk of refractive lensectomy is low. There is a risk of less than one percent that refractive lensectomy may result in intraocular infection, inflammation, bleeding, retinal detachment as well as more rare complications. In the majority of cases, these complications can be treated. In rare cases there could be a loss of sight.

For many people refractive lensectomy may be a better option than laser vision correction due to age, early cataracts, or high corrections. Your eye care provider should be able to answer your questions about this procedure or direct you to someone in your area who has experience with refractive lensectomy.

Thermokeratoplasty

Thermokeratoplasty involves treating precise spots on the cornea with either laser or radiofrequency energy to shrink the peripheral cornea and treat farsightedness (hyperopia). Thermokeratoplasty is a safe and effective procedure, but may take some time to stabilize and may require future treatments.

Thermokeratoplasty is used less frequently than laser vision correction or other non-laser options, but may be a good choice for some people. If you are interested in this option you should ask your eye care provider if there are any ophthalmologists in your area that offer this treatment.

Chapter 13: Alternate (non-laser) Vision Correction Options

Astigmatic Keratotomy

Astigmatic Keratotomy (AK) is the use of relaxing incisions to treat astigmatism. This is not commonly used, except in combination with cataract surgery and refractive lensectomy. Limbal relaxing incision is similar to AK but performed in a more peripheral location on the cornea at the time of cataract surgery.

More recently lens implants have become available which can correct for astigmatism. The use of these lens implants at the time of cataract surgery or refractive lensectomy will reduce the need to perform AK.

Radial Keratotomy

Radial keratotomy (RK) was popular prior to discovery of the excimer laser. It involves radial corneal incisions to flatten the cornea to treat nearsightedness (myopia). Since the advent of excimer laser surgery RK has not been a treatment of choice. RK in some cases has resulted and an unstable correction or consecutive farsightedness. Excimer laser corneal treatments offer superior results and have become the procedures of choice for correction of refractive errors.

Summary

If you are not a candidate for corneal laser vision correction you can ask your eye care provider if you may qualify for a non-laser alternative vision correction. If you do not qualify for any type of vision correction surgery, you should work with your eye care provider to work to optimize you vision with corrective lenses. In some cases glasses or contact lenses are the safest and most effective option.

RESOURCES

Geteyesmart.org:	sponsored by the American Academy of Ophthalmology
Mayoclinic.com:	website for the Mayo Clinic
AAO.org:	American Academy of Ophthalmology website
ASCRS.org:	American Society of Cataract and Refractive Surgery website
FDA.gov:	the US FDA site for information on approved devices and medications
Ncbi.nlm.nih.gov/pubmed:	US National Library of Medicine and the National Institute of Health peer reviewed articles
Westernlasereye.com:	website for Dr. Anderson Penno
Optometrist or Ophthalmologist:	your current eyecare provider is likely to have information about services in your area and can refer you to a local expert in this area.

ABOUT THE AUTHOR

Dr. Anderson Penno performed her first PRK in 1996 and has over a decade of experience in refractive surgery. She has performed thousands of surgeries including PRK, Epi-LASIK, LASIK, and Intra-LASIK. Writing has always been part of her career, and she has co-authored numerous articles, book chapters, and two surgical textbooks.

Dr. Anderson Penno lives and works in Calgary, Alberta, Canada. Her training includes a BS degree from Carleton College in Northfield, MN, an MD and MS from University of Minnesota, ophthalmology residency at the Mayo Clinic in Rochester, MN, and a refractive surgery and research fellowship at the Gimbel Eye Centre in Calgary, AB. More information about Dr. Anderson Penno can be found at www.westernlasereye.com.

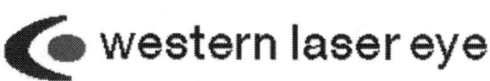

Suite 209, 8555 Scurfield Drive NW
Calgary, AB T3L 1Z6
P: 403.547.9775
F: 403.247.9774

GLOSSARY

Aberrations: variations in the optics of the eye.

Aberrometer: a device that uses infrared light to measure precise variations in the optics of the eye called aberrations. These measurements are used in wavefront treatments.

Ablation: the process of removing corneal tissue with the excimer laser.

Amblyopia: refers to an eye that has reduced vision as a result of developmental issues which limit the ability of the eye to see 20/20. Amblyopia is also called "lazy eye".

Anterior Chamber: the aqueous filled space between the lens of the eye and the cornea.

Aqueous: the fluid in the front part of the eye which is responsible for maintaining the proper pressure inside the eye.

ASA: Advanced Surface Ablation. An acronym used by some people to describe the combination of wavefront treatment and surface no-flap techniques.

AST: Advanced Surface Treatment. An acronym used by some people to describe the combination of wavefront treatment and surface no-flap techniques.

Astigmatism: a term used to describe an optical condition that can result in the need for glasses. Astigmatism usually results from a cornea that is not perfectly spherical but that is shaped more like a basketball. Astigmatism is sometimes due to variations in the lens of the eye.

Bifocal: eye glasses with a visible reading segment in the lower part of the glass.

Blepharitis: a condition related to rosacea that causes plugging of the oil glands along the eyelid margin that causes irritation, dry eye, and redness.

Cataract: a clouding of the lens inside the eye.

Co-Management: a term used to describe an arrangement between two qualified eye care providers where the care of a patient is shared.

Conjunctiva: the outer clear membrane that covers the white part of the eye (sclera).

Consent: the legal document which discusses the possible risks of the surgery you have agreed to have done. Signing this document means you have read and understood the information on the consent.

Cornea: the clear outer layer of the central part of the eye in front of the colored part of the eye (iris). The cornea is analogous to a windshield.

Corneal Dystrophy: conditions which can cause warpage, thinning, or other corneal changes. Corneal dystrophies including keratoconus and pellucid are usually hereditary.

Corneal Mapping: devices which create a topographic map of the corneal surface and in some instances also provide a thickness map and information about the posterior corneal surface.

Cycloplegia: the use of medicated drops to dilate (widen) the pupil. These drops also temporarily paralyze the focusing muscles of the eye.

Cycloplegic Refraction: also called a wet refraction which is a measurement for corrective lenses that is done after drops are instilled to relax the focusing muscles.

Cyclotorsion: rotation of the eye which can occur when supine (lying on your back).

Dilation: a synonym for cycloplegia.

Diopter: an optical unit of measurement used to note the power of corrective lenses.

Dry Refraction: also called a manifest refraction which is a measurement for corrective lenses that is done without drops.

Ectasia: a corneal condition causing thinning and warping of the cornea that in rare cases can occur following laser vision correction or that can be caused by a corneal dystrophy.

Enhancement: a second laser treatment used to refine (touch up) small amounts of residual nearsightedness, farsightedness, or astigmatism after laser vision correction.

Epi-LASIK: a newer type of surface no-flap laser vision correction which uses a device called an epikeratome to re-

Glossary

move the outer surface epithelium of the cornea for laser vision correction.

Epikeratome: a device with an oscillating separator used to prepare the surface of the eye for the laser application during Epi-LASIK.

Epithelium: surface "skin" cells. The corneal epithelium is a thin layer of cells that cover the outer cornea.

Excimer: the specialized type of laser used to precisely remove corneal tissue during laser vision correction surgery.

Eye Tracker: many lasers have a device which will move the location of the laser treatment during the laser firing in order to adjust for small eye movements and stay aligned through out treatment.

Farsighted: the common name for hyperopia which means that the eye must exert focal power to see clearly even at the distance.

Femtosecond: a specialized ultra-fast laser used to create the corneal flap for Intra-LASIK procedures.

Forme Fruste: a term used to describe a corneal dystrophy which is not causing any vision changes. Usually found by corneal mapping in people without vision problems.

Glaucoma: elevated pressure inside the eye and/or damage to the optic nerve resulting in reduced peripheral vision. A variety of conditions can result in glaucoma.

Higher Order Aberrations: optical variations that are more complex than simple nearsightedness, farsightedness, and astigmatism. These aberrations are treated during wavefront laser vision correction surgeries.

Hyperopia: also called farsightedness which describes an eye that must exert focal power even to see clearly at the distance.

ICL®: implantable contact lenses (also called phakic-IOL) used for non-laser vision correction surgery.

Intra-LASIK: the name for the creation of a flap with the femtosecond laser that is used in combination with the excimer laser for laser vision correction.

Intraocular: inside the eye.

IOL: intraocular lens implant used for cataract surgery and for clear lensectomy (refractive lensectomy) which is a non-laser vision correction surgery.

Iridotomy: small holes made in the iris to provide alternate fluid circulation within the eye. Iridotomies may be done for narrow angle glaucoma or to prepare the eye for phakic-IOL implantation

Iris: the colored part of the eye located within the eye just in front of the lens. The iris is analogous to a shutter in a camera and is responsible for pupil size changes.

Iris Recognition: the use of iris landmarks which are unique to every individual to achieve a rotational adjustment during wavefront laser treatments which enhances accuracy.

KASA: Keratome Assisted Surface Ablation. An acronym to describe Epi-LASIK.

Keratoconus: a hereditary corneal dystrophy which in severe cases can lead to corneal irregularities.

Keratometry: measurements of the corneal curvature.

Laser Vision Correction: a common term to describe the use of the excimer laser for surgeries that eliminate or reduce the need for corrective lenses.

LASIK: Laser In Situ Keratomeleusis. A surgery that involves creating a corneal flap with a microkeratome device for laser vision correction.

Macula: the center part of the retina which is responsible for sharp central acuity. The macula is affected in age related macular degeneration (AMD).

Manifest: the term used to describe the measurement of the eye's corrective error which is done without the use of drops. This is sometimes called a dry refraction.

Microkeratome: the device used to create the corneal flap during LASIK surgery.

Monovision: the term used to describe correcting one eye for distance and leaving the other eye nearsighted for reading.

Myopia: the technical name for nearsighted which means that even when the eye is completely relaxed the focal point is closer than infinity.

Glossary

Nearsightedness: the common name for myopia which means that the focal point of the eye is closer than infinity even with the eye fully relaxed.

Opaque Bubble Layer (OBL): a temporary whitening of the cornea which can occur during intra-LASIK surgery.

Ophthalmologist: a medical doctor (M.D.) with a subspecialty in eyes and eye surgery.

Optic Nerve: the largest nerve in the body, the optic nerve is responsible for transmitting the information from the retina to the visual areas of the brain for processing.

Optometrist: a doctor of optometry (O.D.) who is trained in non-surgical care of the eye.

Pachymetry: corneal thickness.

Pellucid Marginal Dystrophy: a hereditary condition that in severe cases can cause irregularities of the cornea.

Photophobia: light sensitivity that can result from many conditions.

Progression: the natural increase in nearsightedness in youth and young adults.

Progressive: also called a line-less bifocal. A lens with a progressively changing prescription from distance at the top to reading or close correction at the bottom.

PRK: Photorefractive Keratectomy. The original no-flap surface laser vision correction technique introduced in North American over twenty years ago in which the surface corneal epithelial cells are removed using a manual method.

Presbyopia: the age relate loss of focusing ability that results in the need for reading glasses, bifocals, or progressive lenses sometime after forty years old.

Ptosis: a drooping of the upper lid that can be caused by a variety of conditions.

Pupil: the black central space in the center of the colored part of the eye (iris). The pupil is black due to the fact that light entering the eye is not ordinarily reflected back out of the eye except in uncommon cases such as the red eye effect with a camera flash.

Refraction: the measurement of the need for corrective lenses.

Refractive surgery: refers to surgeries done to reduce or eliminate the need for glasses or contact lenses; also called laser vision correction if the excimer laser is used.

Regression: a healing response following laser vision correction that shifts the eye back towards the original correction.

Retina: the layer in the back of the eye behind the vitreous which is responsible for receiving images. The retina is analogous to film in a camera.

SBK: Sub-Bowman's Keratomeleusis. A newer LASIK technique which involves creating a very thin corneal flap during LASIK surgery.

Sclera: the white connective tissue the surrounds the entire eye with the exception of the central area which is covered by the clear cornea. The sclera is covered by conjunctiva.

Slit Lamp: a specialized microscope used to examine the eye in the clinic. Often used in combination with specialized lenses to view both the front surface and the interior structures including the central retina.

Strabismus: also known as "squint" or "lazy eye". Refers to an imbalance in the muscles surrounding the eye which can result in a crossed or turned eye.

Technician: the staff that assists ophthalmologists and optometrists with vision measurements and other pre-testing of the eye as well as in some cases patient counseling. Often technicians are certified by JCAHPO.

Toric: astigmatic. Some lenses are toric which means they include a correction for astigmatism.

Vitreous: the gel like substance that fills the back of the eye in front of the retina but behind the lens inside the eye.

Wavefront: refers to methods which involve the measurement of light waves exiting the eye to create a map of higher order aberrations. Wavefront measurements are used to create an individualized correction pattern for use in wavefront laser vision correction.

INDEX

Aberrations: 13, 50, 78, 168, 169
Aberrometer: 25
Ablation: 6, 10, 75, 76, 79
Amblyopia: 89, 118
Anterior Chamber: 99, 111, 112, 161, 175
Aqueous: 99, 100, 111
ASA: 79
AST: 79
Astigmatism: 24, 29, 30, 34, 36, 37, 39, 43, 44, 45, 78, 85, 101, 127, 129, 131, 138, 141, 143, 151, 153, 155, 163, 164, 166, 168, 173, 175, 177
Bifocal: 13, 24, 29, 32-34, 89, 101, 114, 175
Blepharitis: 103, 104, 119, 174
Cataract: 15, 21, 33, 39, 47, 114, 115, 119, 130, 143, 154, 165, 167, 174, 175, 177
Co-Management: 64
Conjunctiva: 99, 106, 107, 136, 147, 159
Consent: 5, 18, 19, 87, 91, 92
Cornea: 5, 6, 12, 30, 36, 44-46, 50, 47-50, 60, 68, 72, 69, 78, 87, 88, 100, 108-111, 119, 120, 138
Corneal Dystrophy: 30, 47, 110, 138
Corneal Mapping: 12, 35, 44-46, 50, 60, 72, 111, 151

Corneal Thickness: 35, 36, 42, 44, 45, 50, 110, 151, 163
Cycloplegic Refraction: 25, 27, 29, 43, 50
Cyclotorsion: 30, 112, 169
Dilation: 25, 27, 90
Diopter: 27, 37, 38, 42, 43
Dry Refraction: 25
Ectasia: 12, 27, 44, 45, 48, 72, 85, 87, 88, 109, 110, 127, 139, 150, 151, 162, 163
Enhancement: 15-18, 30, 37, 40, 84
Epi-LASIK: 8-10, 16, 35, 42, 44, 62, 69-81, 107, 108, 116, 117, 133-143, 144, 151, 162, 168
Epikeratome: 8, 73, 76, 133, 134, 136-138, 143
Epithelium: 44, 62, 76, 108, 109, 110, 126, 127, 133, 134, 137-139, 148, 150, 160, 162
Excimer: 5, 10, 62, 77, 167, 168
Eye Tracker: 122, 134, 146, 148, 158, 160
Farsighted: 15, 24, 28-30, 34, 36, 42, 43, 78, 85, 173, 176, 177
Femtosecond: 9, 10, 21, 63, 73-75, 79, 151, 157, 160, 167, 170, 171
Forme Fruste: 111

Glaucoma: 112, 47, 48, 117-119, 167, 175
Higher Order Aberrations: 13, 78, 168, 169
Hyperopia: 24, 28, 29, 42, 78, 167, 171, 176
ICL: 173, 175
Intra-LASIK: 8, 9, 16, 35, 42, 44, 53, 62, 69-81, 85, 86, 106-110, 116, 117, 151, 158-168, 170, 171
IOL: 173-5
Iris: 5, 30, 49, 77, 99, 100, 111-113, 169, 175
Iris Recognition: 77, 112, 113, 169
KASA: 79
Keratoconus: 30, 44, 45, 47, 48, 50, 51, 72, 87, 111, 119, 120, 151, 163
Keratometry: 50
LASIK: 8-10, 16, 35, 42, 44, 53, 58, 62, 63, 69-81, 85-87, 106-110, 116, 117, 144-155
Macula: 47, 48, 100, 117, 120
Manifest Refraction: 25, 50
Microkeratome: 9, 8, 44, 63, 72-76, 145, 149, 151, 152, 157, 160, 162, 170
Monovision: 33, 38, 39, 41, 70, 89, 114, 118, 176
Myopia: 24, 26, 27, 42, 78, 177
Nearsightedness: 26, 27, 30, 34, 37, 39, 42-44, 78, 101, 168, 174, 177
Ophthalmologist: 6, 18, 20, 54, 56, 59, 64, 80, 89, 90, 117, 176

Optic Nerve: 49, 100, 101, 117-119
Optometrist: 6, 7, 18, 20, 56, 64, 65, 80, 89, 91, 117
Pachymetry: 50
Pellucid Marginal Dystrophy: 44, 45, 47, 48, 111, 119, 120
Progression: 27
Progressive: 13, 24, 29, 32, 33, 37, 114, 120
PRK: 8-10, 16, 20, 35, 42, 44, 53, 58, 62, 63, 69-81, 87, 108, 109, 121-131, 133, 143, 146, 168
Presbyopia: 24
Ptosis: 103
Pupil: 50, 100, 112, 113, 170
Refraction: 23, 24, 25, 27, 29, 35-37, 43, 50, 151, 163
Regression: 29, 125, 127, 128-130, 136, 139, 141, 142, 150, 153, 154, 162, 164, 165
Retina: 24, 47-50, 90, 100, 101, 117, 120, 167, 171, 176
SBK: 63, 72, 74, 79, 151
Sclera: 99, 106-108, 147, 159
Slit Lamp: 30, 50, 90, 92, 111
Strabismus: 120
Technician: 6, 7, 65
Toric: 30, 43, 175
Vitreous: 49, 100, 101, 111, 116, 117
Wavefront: 12, 14, 16, 20, 25, 45, 50, 62, 70, 77-79, 111-114, 168, 169

Made in the USA
Charleston, SC
24 February 2012